T0331775

# AT THE
# HUMAN
# EDGE

### The Limits of Human Physiology
### and Performance

# AT THE HUMAN EDGE

## The Limits of Human Physiology and Performance

**Dr. Marcus Ranney**

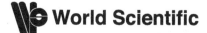
World Scientific

NEW JERSEY · LONDON · SINGAPORE · BEIJING · SHANGHAI · HONG KONG · TAIPEI · CHENNAI · TOKYO

*Published by*

World Scientific Publishing Co. Pte. Ltd.

5 Toh Tuck Link, Singapore 596224

*USA office:* 27 Warren Street, Suite 401-402, Hackensack, NJ 07601

*UK office:* 57 Shelton Street, Covent Garden, London WC2H 9HE

**Library of Congress Cataloging-in-Publication Data**
Names: Ranney, Marcus, author.
Title: At the human edge : the limits of human physiology and performance / Dr. Marcus Ranney.
Description: New Jersey : World Scientific, [2021] | Includes index.
Identifiers: LCCN 2020001693 | ISBN 9789811210112 (hardcover) |
    ISBN 9789811211270 (paperback) | ISBN 9789811210129 (ebook) |
    ISBN 9789811210136 (ebook other)
Subjects: LCSH: Human beings--Effect of environment on--Popular works. |
    Human physiology--Popular works. | Extreme sports--Physiological aspects--
    Popular works. | Extreme environments--Physiological aspects--Popular works.
Classification: LCC QP82 .R425 2021 | DDC 612--dc23
LC record available at https://lccn.loc.gov/2020001693

**British Library Cataloguing-in-Publication Data**
A catalogue record for this book is available from the British Library.

Cover design by Niral Parekh, Studio Amalgamist Inc. (New York).

For photocopying of material in this volume, please pay a copying fee through the Copyright Clearance Center, Inc., 222 Rosewood Drive, Danvers, MA 01923, USA. In this case permission to photocopy is not required from the publisher.

For any available supplementary material, please visit
https://www.worldscientific.com/worldscibooks/10.1142/11545#t=suppl

Printed in Singapore

To my children, Aeden and Eva, who have brought purpose to my biological existence. I hope these words inspire the same passion for science as I have been fortunate to experience.

To my wife Raina, whose relentless support and companionship encourages my ever evolving list of pursuits and allows me to keep dreaming of living life at the human edge.

# Foreword

## by Sir Chris Bonnington
## CVO, CBE, DL, British Explorer

My life has been rich with adventure. The high altitude environment, in which I have spent so many years of my life, is probably one of the most unforgiving and technically challenging on this planet. My first taste of mountaineering began in the winter of 1951 when I hitchhiked to Snowdonia. There, all around me, was adventure. I was excited by the risk and the beauty of the mountains and from that moment I was hooked. In the Himalayas alone I have participated in 19 expeditions, 4 of which were to Everest and for a brief period of time I held the record of being the oldest person to have summited it — aged 50. Climbing is a dangerous game, and climbing at extremes is particularly so.

The South face of Everest is an iconic climb; it's not just the reputation and its story. It is an extraordinary mountaineering test, it has every kind of climbing on it. It's a huge complex face, with so many challenges. There is not a mountain face like it, anywhere in the world. If you overlay this with its history and tragedies — it creates this hugely powerful aura which I think is one of the most unique on our planet.

Each time I went up, and eventually climbing its summit successfully in 1985, I didn't sleep much before, and couldn't help thinking of the stories of those who lost their lives on this mountain. The moment I got on the face, all that vanished and I was completely immersed in the climb itself.

Climbing gives me the biggest buzz I have ever come across. It starts with the physical process of using your body and physiology to get up a stretch of rock; and that in itself is immensely satisfying. Then you build in the element of risk, which is an inherent part of climbing. Fear is an absolutely essential emotion for any climber to stay alive, for fear is actually telling you about the real dangers around you and helps you focus. The important thing is to, having focused the mind, assess how dangerous it is; whether and how to carry on and in helping you concentrate in order to survive. The exhilaration of this process is indescribable.

At the age of 85, I have realized that as you get older, it's important to remember, don't give up. Make life as rich and exciting as you possibly can. Achieving success requires a huge amount of hard work, most of which is boring and dull. Work hard and live life to fulfill your own potential. In reading the words in this book, I hope future scientists, doctors, climbers and adventurers are inspired to push the boundaries of science further, to scale new heights of discovery and summit new peaks of achievement. Creating a better world for the current and future generations. Falling in love with nature and the outdoors and this beautiful gift — the human body.

# Review

## by Jonty Rhodes
## Former International Cricketer
## Current Coach, Commentator, Traveller

*At the Human Edge*, by Dr. Marcus Ranney, is not just a book for elite athletes looking to improve their performances, but a guide for all of us, to journey towards our "best self".

My wife is both a qualified architect and yoga teacher, and what she has demonstrated to me, is the importance of a solid foundation, a functioning structure; and that everything is connected. For our family, this foundation is enhanced through good nutrition and conscious lifestyle choices, which is not about following the latest diet or fitness trend, but more about doing what you love with a body that you honour.

Through yoga and now ayurveda, coupled with the benefits of cold water swimming and other healthy activities, I have crossed the 50 mark without needing to address any health issues. This has been achieved, just like in my playing days, where I was an above average performer on the field, by focusing on the "labour", and not the "fruits" of what this labour might bring me.

Hours of practice and making good decisions in high intensity situations, allowed me to focus on the process, and not entirely on the outcome. This meant that emotional highs were not followed by crashing lows, as long as I honestly believed that I had left "nothing in the tank" in my preparation for the match.

We are constantly evolving and learning, and being open to guidance is important; however, in this fast paced world we live, we really all need to take the time to listen to our body — as it inherently knows what is best for us. And sometimes listening to the body means ignoring the complaints or rather the limitations of the mind.

Dr. Marcus Ranney inspires us to go beyond that limitation and by doing that, to truly be alive and operate at your fullest potential.

# Afterword

## by Dr. Tedros Adhanom Ghebreyesus
## Director General
## World Health Organization

From James Cameron's voyage to the depths of the Mariana Trench to Neil Armstrong's first steps on the moon, Dr. Marcus Ranney paints an intriguing picture of how the human body responds to and what it's capable of under the most extreme conditions.

Advances in physiology, biochemistry, genomics and other areas of science have opened new frontiers for human health. And yet many mysteries remain about how our bodies work, and many challenges to human health are still to be solved. More than ever, we need a new generation of young scientists who will continue to push back the boundaries of the unknown.

But human health does not exist in a vacuum — as the COVID-19 pandemic has demonstrated, it is inextricably linked with the health of our planet through the air we breathe, the water we drink, the food we eat and the conditions in which we live. Any efforts to improve human health must therefore include efforts to protect the earth that sustains us.

In that sense, many of the world's health most pressing health problems are not scientific challenges at all; they are challenges of politics, economics, agriculture, energy, commerce and trade.

Without exception, the extraordinary feats described in this book were accomplished by men and women in good health. This points to a fundamental truth: that health is the foundation for humans to do amazing things. The fact that billions of people globally lack access to the food, water, clean air and health services they need to be healthy is therefore not only a moral outrage, it's a brake on human progress.

Ultimately, ensuring that all people can access the health services they need, without facing financial hardship, is not just the right thing to do, it's a platform for future generations of humans to achieve even more amazing deeds than those described in this book.

# Contents

# Introduction

*"Life is either an incredible adventure, or it is nothing at all."* These words have fascinated me, stirred my soul, and made me want to experience all there is to experience in this world. But alas, even with the most worthy of intentions, the limitations of urban living and day-to-day routines restrict my ability to truly live out this sentiment, as would be the case for many of you too, I'm sure. But fortunately there are individuals amongst us, call them thrill seekers or adventure junkies — the ones who really *do* live life each day to the maximum — who continue to experience the amazing wonders that this planet (and beyond) has to offer. Through their own accounts, they inspire us mere mortals to try and push ourselves just that little bit more each day so that we may, in our little own way, experience what it means to truly live.

Ironically, I was introduced to the world of adventure not through the great outdoors but, believe it or not, from a chemistry textbook instead. It was my third year of study at University College London Medical School and I had taken a year's sabbatical to complete a Bachelor of Science degree in Physiology. Looking through the modules at the start of the year, my eyes lit up when I saw the course 'Space and Extreme Physiology' which was to be conducted by some of the most dynamic and enthusiastic lecturers in the field. I immediately applied for the course and luckily I got in. As I sat there in the lecture halls listening to these legends of physiology speak about their domain expertise and how they did their research at the far-flung corners of the world, a spark was lit in me. As the years progressed, it was this spark that ignited and fueled my passion for research into human physiology and the processes that allow this amazing machine of ours to cope with everything that's thrown at it! And as the years wore on, I found myself in a position to witness the changes, which I had read about in the books and which I shall describe in detail in this book, come alive in front of my very eyes.

Joining the University of London Air Squadron, I enlisted in the Royal Air Force and felt the thrill of flying. Whilst the contents of my stomach revisited me on many occasions I achieved a childhood dream and got to pilot an aeroplane for the first time. Winter training took me to various places across the European Alps as I earnt my ski legs. The greatest honour was working alongside jet pilots and to study the effects of extreme g-forces on their physiologies.

A few years later I found myself leading a hundred-strong team to Mt. Everest. A summer trip, which was meant to be a month long holiday with four friends from medical school, quickly snowballed and became one of the largest medical research expeditions ever to Everest. Almost two years of planning, nearly three tonnes of equipment and a team of 60 student doctors and additional support staff and crew, the August of 2007 was one of the most life changing months in my entire life. I fell in love with oxygen and more importantly the role of mitochondria. For this reason, the penultimate chapter of this book is dedicated to this amazing little cellular organelle, without which life (as we know it) may not have been possible.

The following year, in my final year of medical school, after a brief stint with the helicopter ambulance emergency services in London, I was introduced to an affiliate service provider supporting the International Space Station's transportation system. Some email and phone exchanges later, I found myself settling in to Coco Beach, Florida for a month long internship with the medical team at Kennedy Space Centre, NASA. I literally had to pinch myself!

All the lectures and books I read during my physiology degree suddenly became reality. I felt like I was going to space! My assignment was to support the medical team involved in Mission STS-122, space shuttle Atlantis' space station. On board was the to-be installed science and research module "Columbus" which was built by the European Space Agency. An assignment which was so intimate to the overall mission, my mentors allowed me access to areas unimaginable. The four weeks culminated in being physically present, for the launch of the shuttle, just a few miles away. Feeling its power tear through my body, as the space shuttle roared into the blue sky above me. A few weeks later, in the early hours of the morning, just as dawn broke, I stood off the runway at Kennedy as I watched Atlantis return to earth. A series of sharp 's' turns and the double sonic boom of its fuselage breaking the sound barrier, this flying brick came to a stop a few hundred metres in front of me with its collapsing drone parachutes.

The years went by and I graduated from medical school and practiced in London as a doctor. It was on one of my late night on-calls, as a surgical house officer in north London, that I received a strange email. I almost deleted it. It was an invite to lead a team from Great Britain to participate in an outdoors, winter games festival, being held in the northernmost region of Siberia, deep in the arctic circle. Three months later, rounding up some friends and colleagues (and equipment), we landed in Moscow airport and we made the near four thousand kilometre train journey to Yamalo-Nenets. For a week, in sub zero conditions, we battled against teams from North America and Europe in some of the most isolated and scenically stunning physical environments I could have dreamt of. We used the opportunity of this expedition, to study the effects of the cold weather and extreme physical stress on our bodies.

I was hooked; physiology was my thing. But like for so many of us, life is full of zigs and zags, most of them not under our control at all, and mine did the same. A few years later, cutting a long story short, I decided to chase a girl and move to Mumbai. Leaving the clinical world behind, I now focused my professional attention towards healthcare systems and its management. Fast forwarding to today, more than ten years on, the story has ended up being pretty fantastic. That girl I chased, well she became my wife and marrying her was probably the smartest decision I have ever made!

I now find myself at the unique intersection of health and technology. A niche which I have carved out for myself over the past decade. My fascination has led me from the world of sick-care to healthcare, leveraging the power of digital technology to augment this journey. More than this, the past five years have led me on my own personal journey of wellbeing. Becoming addicted to long distance running, in January of 2020 I completed my first full marathon, a feat which I had dreamt about for almost fifteen years. Pushing my physical fitness as far as I can, I have trained for triathlons, obtained a guiness record (for running backwards) and have thoroughly fallen in love with the discipline. Something which, as you shall read about in the final chapter of this book, has led me to appreciate what the real driving force behind our physical capabilities truly is.

And now, in my late thirties, with two children of my own, I often reminisce of the wonderful opportunities and adventures which I have been afforded through my life. Connecting the dots has been a fascinating experience and it was in one of those deeply contemplative moments which the spark of an idea, to write this book, began. As I obsess each day around human performance, achieving one's peak, optimising for greatness, how did this journey really begin? This is the story of that journey.

Rewinding the clock back, long before my own existence, my ancestor's existence, or even that of primates and mammals. Going back in time to the primordial ooze where life first started, our body has evolved over thousands of generations to excel under the conditions it is constantly exposed to. Every aspect of the environment we take for granted, such as the ambient temperature, the light of the sun, the force of gravity, the composition of the air or the pressure of the atmosphere, are the conditions our evolving bodies have reliably been subjected to for millions of years. And as the years and generations have gone by, our bodies, which first adjusted and then became accustomed to each of these environmental factors, have now become reliant on them for our very own survival.

I would assume that the majority of you are reading this book are doing so in the comforts of an oxygen-rich and moderate temperature environment, all the while being well-hydrated and satiated after a calorie-rich meal and safely protected from the elements by a sturdy mix of concrete, glass and metal. Would I be wrong to think this? And whilst sitting there reading these words, unknowing to you, your body is undergoing thousands of complex biochemical processes in order to do two things for the trillions of cells that have come together to make you up — provide nutrients such as glucose and oxygen in order to manufacture the energy needed by your cells, and remove the harmful waste products that build up in cells, such as toxins, carbon dioxide and various metabolites.

What I find truly amazing is that even though our bodies — these multi-dimensional, energy-producing, waste-removing, organic machines — are engaged in these intricate events while seated in the comforts of our homes or offices, they would continue to do so even if we were transported to the minus 40 degree Celsius environment of the South Pole, the oxygen-depleted 9,000-metre height of Mt. Everest or the bone-crushing, cold depths of the Pacific Ocean. Through a series of rapid physiological and biochemical alterations, the human body can adapt and transform itself to cope remarkably with the harshness of the environment it finds itself in.

When we think about many of the great expeditions throughout history, a lot of which we shall read about together in this book, what immediately comes to your mind? Some of us may think about the technological advances in equipment or vehicles needed for adventurers to reach their destinations. Others may think of their teams, from the brave crew to their dedicated support staff, or the vast quantities of supplies, fuel and consumables that were needed. And of course there's also the eyepopping sums of money required to finance these expeditions. But how many of us think about the bodies of these expeditionists, I wonder? Their amazing physical characteristics that allowed them to complete these superhuman feats of endurance, as well as the internal 'journey' taken by their own physiology in order for these incredible endeavours to be accomplished?

As I look back at my own journey, it is this raw yet elegant power of the human body to adapt and excel that had captured my imagination back in school and which continues to drive me today. This has taken me from reading chemistry textbooks to actually exploring these environments firsthand some years later and analysing the real-time physiological changes of our bodies in such environments. And through this book, its chapters which explore some of the most extreme environments known to man, I hope that my own stories and those of amazing adventurers through history, can act as a backdrop to inspire you to learn more about the human body. I hope to be able to spark a curiosity in each and every one of you like it happened for me, so that the next time you are running the London marathon, scuba diving in the Indian Ocean or skiing in the French Alps or, maybe one day soon (hopefully), be aboard a private spacecraft to orbit earth, you may also have a greater appreciation of the cellular changes happening inside yourself as you pursue life to the fullest!

# 1 Everest

"*Great things are done when men and mountains meet.*"

**— William Blake, Gnomics Verse 1**

*I stood on the lunar-like landscape with my mouth gaping wide open, in awe of the mountain that still towered up, up and up in front of my eyes. For thirteen days we had walked. Day after day, sometimes for ten to twelve hours. Battling the intense rain, the sheer cold, and the thin air. My lungs hurt as the last few hours' climb to reach where I now stood was tough. Even though I knew my body was strong and in better shape than it had ever been, it was still hard. My head felt full and I was unable to tell whether this was due to the altitude sickness or the sheer emotion of finally being here. It was in many ways my moment. I knew that I had achieved something special. From a mere idea more than two years ago to actually making it here, and to do it in such a grand way, was an achievement and one, which I knew, would shape me and my direction in life from this point on. Team Everest, an expedition team a hundred strong and led by me, was one of the largest medical research expeditions in history to reach Mt. Everest's base camp. This was also the first time a student-led expedition had achieved such scale and ability. I found a quiet rock away from the main group and I sat down and paused. I just looked at the mountain and smiled.*

— Personal diary excerpt, expedition journal,
Team Everest 2007

Mountains have captured the human spirit of adventure for centuries. Visually stunning, naturally awesome and unmatched in size and scale, from the ancient Greeks to the modern-day Nepalese, humans have always revered mountains and upheld them as sacred. Thinking of mountains, the word 'Everest' is undoubtedly the one name which, in all our minds, epitomises the heroism and courage displayed by all those who have been brave enough to summit the great mountain and return home alive. Since 1953, after Tenzing Norgay and Sir Edmund Hillary's successful climb, there have been more than four thousand people who have successfully followed in their footsteps. This number already seems like a lot, but now add to this the countless others who have attempted and failed or, worse still, died in vain on her slopes and all of a sudden the numbers reach epidemic proportions. And Everest is just one mountain; there are hundreds of other peaks like it across the globe that claim the lives of many climbers every year.

So what is it about mountains that makes them so treacherous? Yes, a large number of casualties occur secondary to the risks associated with climbing. The near vertical mountain faces, the ice-covered jagged outcrops of rock that propel thousands of feet above the ground, the unpredictable weather, the remote inaccessible locations and the lack of first aid if a disaster were to occur. These all contribute to the problem, but the answer to this question is actually even simpler — it all lies in a diatomic, colourless, odourless, tasteless molecule that exists all around us. Something that we take for granted and yet without which our cells would cease to function in a matter of minutes. It's all about oxygen! The answer reminds me of a phrase an Intensive Care Consultant told me on my first day after I arrived at the wards after graduating as a doctor. Starry eyed and wet behind the ears, he told me something which sums this up perfectly: *"Trust no-one, question everything and give oxygen!"*

So what I hear you ask? What of this oxygen? Some of you will remember, from our school days, that oxygen is a highly reactive element that, at room temperature and pressure, binds with another atom of itself to form dioxygen, a colourless, odourless and tasteless diatomic gas with the formula $O_2$. Oxygen happens to be the third-most abundant element in the universe after hydrogen and helium and is the most abundant element in the Earth's crust. Free oxygen atoms are too chemically reactive to appear on Earth without the photosynthetic action of living organisms, mainly plants, which use the energy in sunlight to produce elemental oxygen from water. Thus $O_2$, as we know it, only really began to appear in our planet's atmosphere after the evolutionary appearance of photosynthetic organisms, roughly 2.5 billion years ago.

Many of the major classes of organic molecules in living organisms, such as proteins, carbohydrates and fats, contain oxygen. And it is also present in many major organic compounds like shells, teeth and bone. If you really think about it, the mass of living organisms mostly comprises oxygen as it is part of water which makes up about two thirds of our bodies! But the main importance of oxygen is that it comprises about 21% of our atmosphere and is the key ingredient in the body's respiratory process (interestingly, when three atoms of oxygen come together, we end up with a highly reactive, poisonous, blue gas called ozone. It's not all bad news though as ozone protects life on Earth by absorbing solar ultraviolet radiation in the upper atmosphere).

Structuring our journey together, in order to understand the impact climbing a mountain can have on our human body, we shall be following in the footsteps of a climber making his way up the sides of Mt. Everest. Along that journey, from landing at Lukla and arriving at Everest Base Camp, through the various high camps, to the Summit, our brave climber shall be walking in the historic path taken by climbing legends dating back to Sir Edmund Hillary. I am sure that there are readers who have picked up this book because they intend to intertwine their own story with that of Everest and through reading these words would like to gain an understanding of what to expect along that route to the summit, both in terms of geography but also in terms of physiology. So lets start that journey and begin at the iconic Everest Base Camp (EBC).

## Base Camp — 5400 m / 17700 ft — pO2 = 52% (of sea level)

Located at the foot of the Khumbu Glacier, EBC is surrounded by some of the most iconic peaks on Earth. Arriving at base camp is like entering a surreal international United Nations pop-up festival, being held in one of the most remote and rugged locations on Earth. Tents, equipment, laptops and satellite mobile phones are plenty (including a local high speed broadband wifi network)! In peak climbing season, which is from March to June, it becomes home to hundreds of climbers, trekkers, support staff and sherpas. Life at EBC is a very odd mix of mundane domestic tasks, challenging logistical problem solving, and the occasional flash of life or death survival.

Water freezes quickly, due to the below zero temperatures, making washing clothes, hair and teeth a frustrating affair. Cooks and support crew prepare a near constant supply of hot meals for climbers preparing their bodies for the once in a lifetime (hopefully) mammoth climb which awaits them. And to ensure that 'city-planning rules' are well adhered to — the Sagarmatha

Pollution Control Committee monitors all the activity of the various teams to uphold basic sanitation standards. Toilet and personal washing tents are erected so that waste can be removed in trash bag-lined barrels; hauled to lower elevations and disposed, and rubbish is collected and removed.

Those who wish to 'glamp' — can; for a fee of course. The most luxurious expeditions provide their climbers with walk in tents, with panoramic viewing galleries, carpeted floors, hot showers, dedicated internet spots, mini-cinemas, bean bags, lounge chairs, yoga mats and wellness rooms.

The air is filled with sounds — of the hive like activity in the various expedition tents to the occasional roar of military helicopters desperately fighting the thin air to stay airborne and reach their critical patient which needs to be evacuated to lower down the mountain. But the sound that stays with you forever is the distant earth shaking one made by the near constant avalanches and landslides coming down the faces of Nuptse, Lho La and Pumori. You close your eyes and pray that it's not crashing down around a member of an expedition team.

EBC is a place of hope, anxiety, frustration, arguments and friendships. The lucky few will experience their life-long dreams fulfilled, others will return home with an unfinished task. Sadly, there will inevitably be a few brave souls who don't get to return home at all.

So how does High Altitude feel at first? To most people it's the feeling of shortness of breath, the rise in respiration, which we face when exposed to the high altitude and thin air. To most people, the word respiration means moving air in and out of our lungs so that we can breathe. Unfortunately, that is not the entire truth (for the budding physiologists amongst you that process is actually called ventilation). Respiration is in fact the process of delivering oxygen molecules to the energy powerhouses in our cells called mitochondria so that it can interact with glucose (the fuel in our body which comes from the food we eat) in order to produce little units of energy called adenosine triphosphate, or ATP for short. Without this process, our cells would stall and die in a matter of minutes and life as we know it would cease.

Over the many millennia of evolution, the human body has created an amazingly complex yet efficient way to make this delivery. The process begins with the two great bellows in our chest, our lungs. Through subconscious changes in the muscles around and below our chest (the thorax), its volume rises and falls. The unsung hero of ventilation is the sheet of muscular tissue that internally separates the lungs from the abdomen — the diaphragm. Its movement is the primary driver of the voluminous changes in our chests; much more important than the contraction of the muscles in our chest walls. As the thoracic volume rises, the relative negative pressure sucks air into our lungs, carrying millions of tiny molecules of oxygen deep into our lung tissue to tiny air sacs called alveoli where the gas exchange occurs. You may all be aware of the big wind pipe in the centre of our chest called the trachea. This trachea divides and subdivides hundreds of times and at the very end of these subdivisions are these tiny air exchange chambers. The beauty of this process is that it takes an organ which is about twelve inches high and has a total volume of a few litres and creates a gas exchange interface that covers the area of two tennis courts when spread out — that's efficiency!

Alveoli are themselves a superb method to allow gas exchange. By being just one cell wide, they bring air into contact with blood vessels and this allows the oxygen molecules to make their way into our bloodstream while letting unwanted carbon dioxide exit. Carbon dioxide is a by-product of the aerobic energy producing reaction within cells and can be viewed as a 'waste' product, which therefore needs to be expelled from the body. It does, however, play numerous important roles in the maintenance of various biochemical processes in the body and we will return to this at different points in the book.

Once diffused into the blood, the oxygen molecules are quickly picked up by the doughnut-shaped red blood cells. These red cells contain hemoglobin, a four-chained protein containing the compound heme, which in turn contains iron (hence the red colour). It is the hemoglobin molecule that is responsible for the shape of red blood cells, giving them their characteristic doughnut shape with a thin center rather than a hole. Hemoglobin readily binds to oxygen and locks them on board its journey around the miles upon miles of blood vessels within our body. A point to note is that red blood cells are not doughnut-shaped by pure luck. This physical structure actually allows it to be the most efficiently shaped cell to carry oxygen around.

Once the oxygen molecules are saddled upon the red doughnuts, they quickly make their way from the lungs to our great pump — the heart. This fist-sized, conical structure weighs around 300 g in an adult human. To me, the heart represents one of the most amazing engineering marvels of the biological world, one that simply dumbfounds us when we think about how it came to be. There are many variations of this circulatory pump throughout the natural world — from a single muscular tube in earthworms, a sequential S-shaped structure in fish, three-chambered pumps in frogs, three-and-a-half chambers in turtles, to the mammalian four-chambered version. One of my favourite embryology lectures at medical school was when we traced the evolution of the human heart through so many of our reptilian and amphibian relatives in its journey to become the version we see beating within our own chests today.

Broadly divided into four chambers, the heart's upper two chambers, called atria, receive blood into itself and the bottom two chambers, known as ventricles, are thicker walled — enough to pump blood either to the lungs (for the gaseous exchange of oxygen and carbon dioxide) or around the body. The human heart has a large septum which divides the heart into two halves, with the right side receiving and expelling de-oxygenated blood from the body and to the lungs respectively, and the left side receiving and expelling oxygenated blood from the lungs and to the body respectively. The health of this one-way circuit of blood is maintained by valves. The heart is effectively a syncytium, a multinucleate cell that results from multiple cell fusions of unicellular cells, using an electrical messaging system to control the complex yet efficient circulatory system. We shall delve into the amazingly complex exchanges within the heart in the later chapters of this book.

Roughly beating more than 2 billion times over our lifetime, the heart has an incredible ability to not only alter the frequency of its beat, otherwise known as the heart rate, but it can also alter the actual volume of blood that is pumped out in every beat, something we call stroke volume. By changing these two functional capabilities, our body is able to increase or decrease our cardiac output as required and adjust the amount of oxygen pushed out of the chest to reach the many trillions of cells in our tissues. Effects which, as we shall see in this chapter, are altered as a climber ascends up the slopes of Everest.

## Khumbu Icefall — 5800 m/ 19000 ft — pO2 = 50% (of sea level)

The Khumbu Icefall is located at the head of the Khumbu Glacier and the foot of the Western Cwm and considered to be one of the most dangerous stages of the South Col route to Mt. Everest's summit. As the Khumbu glacier moves down the mountain by 3 to 4 feet every day, the constant movement, along with fluctuating temperatures lead to giant crevasses opening up with no warning and massive seracs (ice towers) tumbling down from over head, their sizes ranging from cars to large houses.

I have heard this part of the route described as a huge horror-chamber at an amusement park. Only this one is for real. Most climbers aim to spend as little time as possible in this stretch, traversing it in the early hours of the morning when the ice is still hard. The constant movement of the glacier under foot means that the terrain is constantly in flux and any ropes and ladders fixed (to help climbers bridge a crevasse) are themselves subject to instability and collapse from movement overnight.

To the unacclimatised, the route can take anywhere between 8 to 10 hours to cross and as most climbing teams prepare an acclimatization schedule by repeatedly moving up and down the mountain; during their 6 to 8 week period of time on Everest, a typical climber may need to traverse this dangerous Icefall at least six times; covering a cumulative distance of almost 25 kilometres in this dangerous terrain.

Whilst dangerous, this distance is dwarfed in relative comparison to the 100,000 kilometres of blood vessels in our body. Laying them all out end to end, they would snake their way across the planet twice — that sure is a lot of distance to cover! Propelled by the cardiac output of our heart, these red cells make their way to all the various organs in our body. Once again dividing and subdividing thousands of times, the vessels become smaller and smaller until they become known as capillaries which embed themselves deep inside our organs. Once again, the reason for doing this is simple. It creates an environment with the smallest possible distance for the oxygen molecules to swim across in order to enter our cells and make their way into the little sausage-shaped powerhouse centres of our cells, the mitochondria. These little furnaces use the broken down sugars such as glucose and mix them together with the highly reactive oxygen molecules to catalyse tiny controlled reactions that release energy, a process called respiration. The energy released is in the form of ATP which all our cells utilise to power our bodies to complete the different activities we want to achieve, which in the case of Everest, would be to climb a mountain!

The process of aerobic respiration, occurring in the presence of oxygen, is significantly more productive than anaerobic respiration in terms of energy. Substances such as carbohydrates, fats, and proteins are consumed as reactants and are first broken down by glycolysis followed by the Krebs cycle and finally the electron transport chain, in a process called oxidative phosphorylation. Most school textbooks state that 38 ATP molecules are made per oxidised glucose molecule during this process of cellular respiration (2 from glycolysis, 2 from the Krebs cycle, and about 34 from the electron transport system). However, this theoretical maximum yield is never quite reached because of leaky membranes as well as the cost of actually moving molecules around the mitochondrial matrix. As such, it is much more likely that around 29 to 30 useful ATP molecules per glucose molecule are actually created.

All in all, the process we have just described is called the oxygen cascade and it captures the journey that molecules must make along the body in order to generate energy. Put another way, it describes the process of the declining oxygen tension from the atmosphere to the mitochondria. Being a gas, the concentration of oxygen through this journey can be represented by its pressure. As we shall see later on, the pressure of oxygen at sea level is 21%

of the standing atmospheric pressure which equates to its concentration, or its partial pressure (PO) to 159 mm Hg (millimetres of mercury — a standard unit of pressure). The first obstacle that oxygen encounters is water vapour, which humidifies inspired air and dilutes the amount of oxygen available to 148 mm Hg. As the air then moves into the alveoli, it is further diluted by carbon dioxide present in the air being expired, which reduces the PO to 100 mm Hg. This is the starting point of oxygen as it enters the bloodstream; as one moves down through the vessels to the cell, the concentration of oxygen is diluted, extracted, or otherwise lost so that the PO may only be 3 or 4 mm Hg at cellular level.

You can perhaps begin to see why this journey — this cascade — is so important. Any small change in the diffusion capabilities at any of the various surfaces involved, in the multiple exchange interfaces that the oxygen molecules encounter from the air to the mitochondria, can have a profound effect on the physical capabilities of the individual. But what is it about climbing mountains that can stir the imagination of a scientist? Why would a doctor be interested in high altitudes?

## Camp I, Valley of Silence — 6100 m / 20000 ft — pO2 = 48% (of sea level)

Just above the Icefall, climbers are greeted to a respite as they enter a flat, almost endless snow-field. Marked by numerous laterally running crevasses (to which you cant see the bottom of) Camp I marks a spot where climbing teams can rest and acclimatise themselves on their summit journey. The bowl shape of the Western Cwm protects the carved out valley from the wind and the valley's snow covered sides reflect the sun, almost amplifying the already intense solar radiation which is already acute at this altitude. Both of these factors can therefore result in climbers being subjected to temperatures as high as 35 degrees celsius — a stark world of a difference from what they were used to at EBC; but which quickly drops to below freezing once the sun drops below the horizon.

This windless, sheltered site is affectionately known as the Valley of Silence. Ironic as the night is filled with deep, murmuring cracking sounds as the ice moves and cracks deep in the glacier beneath, along with plentiful avalanches from the near constant fluctuating temperatures.

Climbers sleep anxiously, hoping that the snow beneath them doesn't suddenly open up a crevasse. And by now, the thin air and resulting hypoxia leads to low grade constant pounding headaches. But through this pain, discomfort and anxiety, for the first time on this treacherous route, a climber taking just a few steps around the corner, will gain his or her first close sight of Everest.

A person may be forgiven for thinking that the main challenge faced by the human body whilst climbing Everest is the sheer intensity of the exercise involved in the climbing process. After all, hauling your body up a ninety-degree face on a piece of rope is no joke. Of course, there is some truth in this, but it is not the whole truth. What we sometimes don't see is the mountaineer who is unable to walk in a straight line on a nearly flat surface at 15,000 feet, or the climber who can barely catch his breath after bending over to tie his boot laces at 26,000 feet. What is it about the environment that can cause this? The answer is a simple one: its technical term is known as hypobaric hypoxia.

Our atmosphere is an ocean of air in which we at sea level inhabit the very depths. Made up of many different gases including oxygen, nitrogen, and carbon dioxide, the 'weight' of the gases in the upper regions of the atmosphere pushes down on the lower layers. This weight generates what is known as atmospheric pressure, which at sea level equates to a pressure reading of 760 mm Hg (while the corresponding pressure of oxygen that is in the inspired air is 148 mm Hg). You can think of this pressure as the effective force at which oxygen is pushed into our bodies, or alternatively the concentration of oxygen in the air.

As we move up through the atmosphere, such as when we are climbing mountains, there is a lower proportion of weight pushing down on us at high altitudes compared to sea level and thus the pressure falls. As this pressure falls, the pressure available to drive oxygen into our bodies also reduces. Oxygen, as I've already mentioned, is our life line. Each cell in our body depends upon it to survive. Without it we can't eat, sleep, run, laugh or think. We can't do whatever it means to be human. Put simply, we can't live without oxygen! Hence it is this reduction in the concentration of oxygen in the air known as hypoxia which results in many of the adverse effects that we see happening to the human body. Taking Mt. Everest as an example, the atmospheric pressure at its summit is 253 mm Hg, which is a third less than it is at the base. But most importantly, the $PiO_2$ (pressure of oxygen in the inspired air) falls to a value of 43 mm Hg! A value that we would consider to be nearly incompatible with life. One of the most amazing things about this value is that it has been estimated that if Mt. Everest was any higher than it currently is, the human body would be totally incapable of climbing it without the use of supplementary oxygen. This is truly one of the many cosmic coincidences that feature in the natural world around us.

My first exposure to high altitude was on a skiing trip in the German Alps. We drove from our hotel in the picturesque town of Oberammergau, which was located at a height of around 900 metres above sea level, up into the hills until we reached the bottom of a cable car station. After boarding the car and through a series of rides, we were shot hundreds of metres up to a ski resort nestled at a height of 2,400 metres. Within twenty to thirty minutes of reaching the resort I began to feel a little bit faint and over the next few hours became increasingly nauseated and generally unwell. This was my first experience of Acute Mountain Sickness (AMS).

AMS afflicts millions of people each year who journey up to high altitudes, typically over 2,400 metres. A series of non-specific symptoms which essentially feel like a hangover after a night of heavy alcohol, AMS is the body's immediate reaction to oxygen scarce environments. This condition is nothing new. The Chinese first documented the ill effects of high altitude in a text written around 37 B.C. which captured the journey of some travelers from China to what is thought to be modern day Afghanistan: "*Again on passing the Great Headache Mountain, the Little Headache Mountain, the Red Land and Fever Slope, men's bodies became feverish, they lose colour and are attacked with headaches and vomiting; the asses and the cattle all being like in condition.*"

AMS typically affects about half of all 'low-landers' who make their way up to high altitude and unfortunately there is no definitive way to predict whether a person will succumb to it or not. Studies have ironically shown that the incidence and severity of symptoms are inversely related to how fit you are. A burley ultra-marathon runner may succumb to its effects whereas a frail 60 year-old woman may find herself completely unaffected. The first feeling one gets is a sense of lightheadedness, as if you were drunk. This then leads into a low-grade headache and general tiredness which makes it hard to walk or want to perform any kind of activity. Some people can find themselves feeling dizzy and short of breath. Sleeping at high altitude is also a suffocating experience where one frequently wakes up in the night gasping for air.

For those who suffer particularly badly, the accompanying nausea can lead a loss of appetite and sometimes vomiting.

The symptoms kick in a few hours after reaching high altitude and most people are able to acclimatise within a day or two. What is interesting to note is that there is no clear long term protection against AMS, even after repeated exposure to high altitude. Whilst a regular climber may be aware of how their body would respond, they are not able to say with absolute certainty that they would not respond badly, even having done the same climb on multiple occasions. What is protective, for lay people and hobbyists, is sticking to the recommended ascent profile along a route. Generally speaking this is to ascend a total of no more than 300 metres in a given day and to build in a rest day (stay at the same altitude) every fourth night.

This process of acclimatisation becomes harder the higher up one goes and any ascent above 7800 metres is deemed dangerous and the body is simply unable to adapt to the conditions. Climbers call this altitude the *'death zone'* and aim to spend as little time as possible in any altitude above this level. In many ways AMS is the body's way of protecting itself from some of the more severe consequences of exposure to high altitude. Two life threatening conditions that can develop within a matter of hours and if not treated immediately, often by returning down to a lower altitude, can quickly lead to death — these are *High Altitude Pulmonary Oedema (HAPE)* and *High Altitude Cerebral Oedema (HACE)*.

## Camp II — 6400 m / 21000 ft — pO2 = 46% (of sea level)

After the ghost like walk, through the silent valley, Camp II (also known as Advanced Base Camp) is a rocky patch which sits at the foot of the icy Lhotse wall. The area is littered with abandoned gear from previous expeditions too fatigued to carry the equipment home, and climbers often spend their time here acclimatising by walking as much as they can, around this area, looking for cool old climbing gear; left here by all of Everest's climbing history.

The location of this camp is absolutely stunning. It's altitude and location means that clouds roll in from the lower ranges of the Himalayas, up the valley and into the camp. And right in front of the climbers lies the dramatic Lhotse Face. Mt. Lhotse, the fourth highest mountain in the world, lies to the right above Camp II and rises to 8,516 metres (27,940 ft); growing from the Mt. Everest massif itself. A magical site, who's peak marks the official border between Nepal, China and Tibet, it is believed that fewer than 400 people have climbed it.

Climbers admiring the stunning views also spend time having their last hot prepared meals on their journey as from this point on they will be surviving on 'instant meals' only. Climbers are now, and for the rest of the climb, in avalanche territory and this will be one of the cautions they will deeply consider every time they place their tents for rest or shelter from the weather.

Combatting the increasingly difficult physical challenges, and now certain AMS, the climber will now face the very real risk of it developing into either HAPE or HACE. And whilst, the exact pathology behind the process of developing AMS is not fully understood, the scientific community largely believes that changes in the permeability of our blood vessels due to the body reacting to low oxygen and increases in blood acidity account for this condition. This change in permeability causes fluids to move across the body more easily, often to places where they shouldn't be. The result is HAPE where there is fluid accumulation in the lungs and HACE which is due to an increase in fluid around the brain.

Pulmonary oedema results from the reaction of the blood vessels in our lungs to the low oxygen. Remember the tiny gas exchanges in the alveoli? At sea level, when there is a reduction in the oxygen delivery capacity of one of these air sacs, the body begins to divert blood away from them to other parts of the lungs so that the most efficient transfer of oxygen can occur. This blood diversion is brought about by squeezing the vessels supplying the alveoli, which then raises the pressure. Under normal circumstances, this increased pressure has no harmful consequences. At high altitudes however, as the overall oxygen level in the air is low, almost all of these alveolar exchanges have low concentrations of oxygen. The body then reacts by constricting the blood flow across all these units. As the sensitivity of this effect is not universally equal, inevitably there are areas where a lot of constriction occurs and other areas where this occurs less. In those areas of the lung where less constriction occurs, the high pressure created in the other areas causes fluid to leak out of the vessels into the lung tissue and this further hinders gas exchange, leading to the symptoms associated with pulmonary oedema.

As the fluid builds up in the lung tissue, climbers become increasingly lethargic and short of breath. The otherwise dry cough that sometimes accompanies the thin crisp air of higher altitudes can turn into a 'wetter' version with sufferers frequently producing copious amounts of sputum. Due to the breakdown of the tiny capillaries, the sputum becomes blood tinged, thereby giving it a slightly pinkish hue. As climbers become increasingly breathless, their rate of breathing and heartbeat begins to rise rapidly and they start to experience tightness in the chest and an inability to catch their breath, particularly whilst lying down. Unfortunately, without the necessary descent to a lower altitude, the delivery of oxygen gas and medications, or the use of a high pressure 'Gamow' bag, which is an inflatable high pressure chamber that can accommodate a single patient, climbers quickly deteriorate to an irreversible stage.

## Camp III, Lhotse Wall — 6800 m / 22300 ft — pO2 = 44% (of sea level)

The Lhotse Face is a 1125 metre (3,690 ft.) high wall of blue glacial ice. One which needs to be scaled head on in one of the toughest environments on the planet. To climb this steep ice face climbers use a device called a jumar, a type of locking carabiner that can free-rise, but then locks onto the rope during the downward motion, so the climbers can effectively pull themselves up using the rope for support. Progress is slow, owing to the hypoxia, treacherous conditions and difficult routine.

After an hour or so of climbing, climbers reach the 'Ice bulge', an icy, bumpy part. The dangerous part is to hang on to the old ropes (of dubious strength) and to change carabiners between the ropes. Made especially trickier as climbers don't feel too clear in their heads. But it's crucial to concentrate, one slip, or wrong clip of the carabiner and the climber plunders hundreds of metres to their deaths, as many do each year.

The climb up the Lhotse face will be either easy or hard, depending on the weather that year. A dry, cold season means sheer, blue ice, requiring a more strenuous crampon kick to fix one's feet. Deep snow however makes the climb easier, but increases the risk of an avalanche.

Climbers then make their way to Camp III, a true eagle's nest, placed right out of the wall — a small ledge on the Lhotse rock face at 7,470 m (24,500 ft). Actually, Camp III is pretty much any spot flat enough that a climber can pitch their tent (thus there are many 'Camp III's'). The space is so small, maybe 150 feet if lucky, and the face so steep, that climbers would never chose to stay here if it weren't for the sheer exhaustion and thin air, and are constantly connected to the safety lines during their time here.

Going to the toilet at night is a tedious task to dress and secure oneself. In addition, just finding a spot for it on this narrow platform is tricky enough. But once done, this toilet provides for one of the best views on Earth.

From Camp III, the climbers continue to traverse the ice wall towards the Yellow Band, a landmark ridge visible between the peaks of Everest and Lhotse. This band is made up of metamorphic rocks, including epidote containing marble, which weathers into a yellowish tone (hence the name). More interesting is the fact that marine fossils have actually been found embedded in this section, which meant that at one point in Earth's history, this part of Everest was actually on the seafloor and confirms the theory of how the Himalayan range was created — by the tectonic plate of the Indian Sub-continent literally slamming into Asia and pushing the two edges up into this majestic natural creation. But at 25,000 feet and after weeks of climbing, understandably no climber has the stamina to look for fossils as we carefully cross this rocky section.

Above the Yellow Band climbers approach the Geneva Spur, an outcropping just below Camp IV. Whilst only a snow field, climbers need to be prepared for dangerously high winds, and scorching temperatures from the sun radiating off the snow and the ever-present risk of avalanches. The day's work, of going from Camp III to Camp IV, is just around 500 metres but one of the most physically demanding routes the climbers will face on this journey.

In December of 2010, the tennis star and 18 times Grand Slam champion Martina Navratilova was hospitalised with high-altitude pulmonary oedema after attempting to climb Mt. Kiliman-jaro, Africa's highest peak (5895 metres). Being 54 years old at the time and still in incredibly great shape, the tennis star was in a 30 member-strong group hiking to the summit for a charity fundraising trip. The tennis pro had never climbed more than 12,000 feet and when she reached 14,800 feet, she began to feel unwell. She later told news reporters that she was 'petrified' of not reaching the summit 'because then the whole world will know.' The trip's accompanying doctor later said, "[She] was feeling more shortness of breath, more breathing issues and seemed to be having a more difficult time than her colleagues. The third night, I was beginning to hear rattling in the lungs and the fluid."

In another case of a fit 28 year-old male Swiss climber to Denali, the examining doctor reported that the patient went to the medical camp on the third day of the expedition (at 4,200 metres) complaining of shortness of breath at rest, a productive cough with pink frothy sputum and an inability to sleep. On closer physical examination, the climber had a pulse of 111 bpm, a respiratory rate of 20 breaths per minute and an arterial oxygen saturation of 74% as measured by a digital pulse oximetre. Furthermore, he was centrally cyanosed (literally blue around the lips, tongue and face) and had bilateral inspiratory crackles upon chest auscultation. The next morning, when a fibreoptic camera tube was inserted down the patient's windpipe and a fluid sample was collected (a bronchoalveolar lavage), the resulting examination of the fluid revealed a blood-stained liquid with an increased number of proteins and white blood cells. This suggested the underlying pathophysiological mechanism of a leaky membrane structure and tissue damage, leading to bleeding and an immune response.

The second life threatening condition that plagues climbers exposed to high altitude is known as HACE. The brain, being the seat of human consciousness and cognitive function, has an unusually large requirement for glucose and oxygen compared to the other major organs in our bodies. Representing only around 2% of our body weight, it guzzles in the region of 20% of our oxygen requirements at rest. For the body to meet the brain's needs, we evolved some very clever mechanisms to protect the blood flow to the brain when our body is starved of oxygen — for example when exposed to high altitude. One way this is done is to increase the amount of blood reaching the grey and white matter of the brain by dilating the tiny blood vessels around it when they 'sense' a reduction of blood oxygen concentration. The body does this because under normal atmospheric conditions, increasing blood flow would automatically increase the number of oxygen molecules being delivered to that region. The resulting increased pressure, which is very similar to the effect we saw in the lungs leading to pulmonary oedema, causes fluid to be pushed out into the space around the brain, leading to the resultant swelling. Along with this physical mechanism, studies have also suggested that there are changes in the hormones and chemicals within the blood vessels in the skull, including inflammation-promoting substances such as nitric oxide and prostacyclin which affect the brain's protective layer known as the blood brain barrier. This changes the structure of the vessels making them more 'leaky' and allowing more fluid to collect in parts of the brain where this shouldn't normally be happening. As the brain sits within the skull and is unable to expand beyond a certain point, this increased pressure can ultimately lead to the brain 'coning' through the base of the skull into the spinal cord and cause the climber to die.

One of the best-known accounts of this condition was beautifully captured in the bestselling book *Into Thin Air* by Jon Krakauer. The author found himself stranded high up on the slopes of Mt. Everest in the catastrophic storm of 1996, one of the worst on record. He describes the effects of HACE on Dale Kruse, a 44 year-old dentist: *"Kruse was having an incredibly difficult time simply trying to dress himself. He put his climbing harness on inside out, threaded it through the fly of his wind suit, and failed to fasten the buckle; fortunately, Fisher and Neal Beidleman noticed the screw up before Kruse started to descend. "If he'd tried to rappel down the ropes like that," says Beidleman, "he would have immediately popped out of his harness and fallen to the bottom of the Lhotse Face." "It was like I was very drunk," Kruse recollects. "I couldn't walk without stumbling, and completely lost the ability to think or speak. It was a really strange feeling. I'd have some word in my mind, but I couldn't figure out how to bring it to my lips. So Scott and Neal had to get me dressed and make sure my harness was on correctly, then Scott lowered me down the fixed ropes." By the time Kruse arrived in Base Camp, he says, "it was still another three or four days before I could walk from my tent to the mess tent without stumbling all over the place."*

The symptoms begin very similar to AMS and this can sometimes be disastrous as climbers think they are suffering from this less potent illness. The headaches worsen and climbers become increasingly confused and imbalanced. Lethargy sets in and the subject develops a feeling of wanting to just lie down and not do anything, regardless of their necessity for survival, which is really dangerous given the circumstances. Fever and unconsciousness soon follow, which can ultimately lead to neurological physical symptoms such as blurred vision and changes in muscle reflexes, breathing and heart rate, ultimately leading to death. It is estimated that there are over 200 dead bodies, almost perfectly preserved by snow and ice, along the upper slopes of Mt. Everest. Many are believed to have succumbed to the fatal effects of HACE as their drive to reach the summit overcame the rational decision to turn back and go home.

In 2007 I led a 100-strong medical research expedition to Mt. Everest base camp. Spending three weeks on the trail up to 5,500 metres, we used ourselves as guinea pigs to measure and quantify the various changes in human physiology that occur as our bodies adapted to the new environment, one without the usual supply of oxygen we are used to. The purpose of this exercise was more than a merely academic one and the results would benefit more than just healthy adventurists who climb, trek or ski at high altitudes every year. There are patients who are fighting for survival every day of the year in every corner of the globe. With physiological systems that have been afflicted and turned inside out by major illnesses, these patients battle to maintain their blood oxygenation against the odds, in particular those who are on critical and intensive care units across the world. If I asked you to picture a patient under intensive care, you no doubt will think of one with tubes and lines entering pretty much any and every orifice in the human body, as well as the main tube supplying oxygen to the patient's lungs, known as the endotracheal intubation tube. This tube is connected to a ventilator machine and its purpose is to do the breathing for the patient as they often cannot do so themselves. And whilst the skilled team of intensivists try to match the rate of breathing and the pressure of air being delivered with each breath, something that continues to trouble doctors is achieving the right amount of oxygen to supply to a patient, as ironically patients who receive high doses of oxygen can fare worse than those who are administered a lower concentration. What doctors are beginning to understand is that while the body is fighting against the oxygen deficiency, either due to a lung infection or a poorly functioning heart and circulatory system, these patients may have adapted themselves to lower oxygen requirements. Therefore, supplying them with more oxygen than needed inadvertently ends up doing more harm than good. As it is difficult to study these adaptive processes in sick patients, a more effective and standardised way to do so is to rely on healthy volunteers, and nature provides no better platform for a low oxygen environment than being at high altitude. With this in mind, studies have been conducted for years by scientists and doctors who push themselves and their peers to these remote yet scenic mountainscapes to study the physiological mechanisms driving these adaptive processes — exactly as we did in that August of 2007.

## Camp IV, the Death Zone — 8000 m / 26000 ft — pO2 = 37% (of sea level)

Camp IV sits on a plateau resembling a moonscape. The air being so thin now that the sky owns a strange, dark blue color; almost like being on the edge of space. A small climb above camp, and climbers can look down the Tibetan plateau — with it's vast brown plains, white glaciers and the other Himalayan giants — Kanchenjunga, Lhotse, Makalu, and sit in awe and wonder of the scenery which surrounds them.

Because of the combined dangers and the disorienting effect at the altitude, the area is known as the Death Zone. The human body is literally dying, at this altitude, and every minute spent here is a race towards death. Climbers can only endure the altitude above Camp IV for a maximum of two or three days. If the weather does not cooperate within that window, climbers are forced to descend.

This is also now the place where the fun and excitement of climbing this mountain becomes a distant memory. All that remains is the harsh reality of the extremely dangerous environment the climber finds themselves in and the knowledge that death can come at any time; and has done to many. The slopes are now littered with bodies of frozen climbers unsuccessful in their summit bids, unlucky on their dreams. A stark reminder of family and friends waiting back home for the climbers' safe return.

People don't talk a lot; preferring instead to rest in their tents. Ensuring that their gear is neatly arranged and prepared for the next day, climbers drink plenty of warm fluids. And as the sun falls, and the winds pick up, they climb clumsily into their tents feeling exhausted and weak already, and try to get some sleep although knowing that they won't get a single wink. For in a couple of hours they will start to put on their gear for the final part of their lifelong adventure — the summit push.

With the climber's oxygen now approaching its lowest, his pulse its highest, it is in the main blood vessels in the neck near a bifurcation that is quite close to where he can feel his pulse where a small group of highly specialised cells called the carotid body chemoreceptors is located. This cluster of cells is adapted to measure the beat by beat changes in the oxygen concentration of the blood flowing past and if they detect the concentration as being too low, a message is fired to the breathing centre in the brain to increase the breathing rate. As the rate increases, we pull in more oxygen from the air, but as a consequence we also end up expelling more carbon dioxide. This paradoxically reduces the drive to breathe and thus limits the maximal rate. Carbon dioxide is a naturally acidic substance and when there is less of it in our blood stream, the alkalinity of the blood increases which is the main inhibitor of our breathing rate. To counteract this mechanism, a longer term and elegantly adaptive response is kickstarted by our kidneys as they begin to expel more alkaline molecules from our blood than normal. This allows a natural equilibrium to be reached whereby the normal ventilator settings of our physiology can be restored. Once again, this reflects a beautiful self-adaptive mechanism that we have evolved over time!

The heart also has a role to play in the body's adaptation to high altitude. It begins by simply increasing the frequency of beats, allowing more blood to be pumped around the body every minute.

To protect itself from low levels of oxygen, it also reduces the stroke volume, which as we have described earlier is the amount of blood pumped out per beat. By doing so, it reduces its own requirement for oxygen, thereby protecting itself from a potentially catastrophic event. Blood begins to redistribute through the many miles of blood vessels in our body as the brain reallocates blood to areas that need it most. More blood flows to the lungs under increased pressure which promotes gas exchange, whereas less blood flows to our 30 feet-long gastrointestinal tract!

## The Summit 8850 m / 29035 ft — $pO_2$ = 33% (of sea level)

Finally, the hour comes, and typically, at around 11 PM the climbers put on their final gear and step out in the night. There, snaking ahead of them in the distance, is a worm of lights slowly moving up a dark wall. The lights are the head torches of other climbers, also making their up this historic path enroute to destiny.

The air is completely silent and nobody dare talks. The atmosphere is absolutely terrifying and the climbers soldier on, higher and higher, awaiting the first rays of sunlight on this new day. It's cold, steep and very icy. The ice axe and crampons, which are now extensions of the climbers body and crucial to survival, barely cut into the ice.

The amazing wonder of the physical universe surrounds the climbers as the Moon rises from below them now and the deep dark expanse of the Milky Way stretches as far as the eye can see over head. But for most climbers, its head down, one foot in front of the other and breathe. Hands freeze, feet freeze, everything freezes. Then finally, after what probably seems like a lifetime of nights, the thin orange hue makes it way over the horizon and the first light of sunrise steps forth.

For those lucky enough to remember to catch it, they are treated to the fabled mountain ghost. The shadow of Everest projects itself onto the morning fog below and towers in front of the climber like a giant triangular mirage. Beneath them now lies the entire world, everything and everyone they love and care about. Above them, a few passenger jets, the International Space Station and who knows what else!

The climbers now reach the Balcony. A good point to have a short rest and change oxygen bottles. A small ridge then lays ahead, called the South Summit. A small plateau of rock, at this point climber's feel like the end is within site — because it is. Just around the corner is the Everest summit itself and hope brings with it the possibility of success, barely 100 metres away, but still at least two hours of climb left to go!

By now climbers have stopped, turned back or worse still fallen to their deaths. And there is one more obstacle in your way. Called The Knife Ridge it is a Cornice Traverse which is the most exposed section of the climb. The boundary between Nepal and Tibet, to its immediate left is a 2,400 metre (8000 ft.) drop down the Southwest Face and to its immediate right is a 3,050 metre (10000 ft.) fall down the Kangshung Face. Certain death on either side and the infamous Hillary Step somewhere in the middle. A rock climb in the sky, it is perhaps nature's last true test to deem whether a climber is worthy of this coveted prize.

It is one of the planet's most well known outcrops of rock and is described as a nearly vertical rock face on Mt. Everest. With a height of around 12 metres and located at an altitude of 8,790 metres (just 60 metres below the summit), the Hillary Step is the last major obstacle to overcome before reaching the highest place on Earth. Putting aside the almost traffic-like congestion on this restricted rock face due to the ever growing volume of climbers during climbing season, at such an altitude it represents a significant physical challenge for the climber to haul themselves, their packs and cylinders, over this technically difficult climbing obstacle. Without factoring in the extreme weather, poor physical conditions for the climbers and significant hypoxia, climbing a nearly vertical 40 feet wall is hard enough as it is. Interestingly in 2017, it was rumoured that the step had collapsed under its own weight, but reports since then and an official statement from the Nepalese Tourism Board have confirmed that this is not true and that while a large rock has indeed broken off, it has merely been covered with a significant amount of snow, giving it a slope-like appearance. What makes this physical obstacle even more daunting is the fact that our physiological ability to maximally exert ourselves reduces drastically as we ascend higher. At altitudes above 1,600 metres, there is an approximate reduction in maximal oxygen uptake of around 8–11% for every 1,000 metres that one climbs. Proponents of utilisation theory for this effect hold that the body's aerobic capacity is limited by a lack of sufficient oxidative enzymes within the cell's mitochondria, whereas those who favour presentation theory argue that our aerobic capacity is instead limited by the ability of one's cardiovascular system to deliver the reduced available oxygen to active tissues. As we have read, it is likely that a combination of both effects contribute to this reduced ability to perform at maximum capacity. Maybe the Hillary Step is just Mother Nature's way of testing the climber one last time before they reach their dream!

After the step, climbers see in front of them a small spot of white, strange wave-like formations, of frozen snow pointing out from the summit. They climb towards this section, usually unroped, but using their axe. It seems to go on and on, fueling frustration and tiredness. But walking on, their destiny in front of them, with the bright blue sky behind is the dream which every climber and perhaps every person has thought of — the summit of Mt. Everest.

Our bodies will never be able to acclimatize to the conditions above 8,000 metres. No amount of physical conditioning or preparation will enable a person to spend more than 48 hours in the Death Zone. The oxygen is barely one third of the pressure at sea level; and we are literally burning it faster than we can replace it. Even with the use of supplemental oxygen via tanks it feels like being choked. In such conditions taking most climbers up to 12 hours to walk the final 1.72 kilometres (1 mile) from the South Col to the summit.

What lays in wait for the successful climber is a small mound of flags and material, something which at sea level could easily be mistaken for a pile of trash. But in those fibres lay the hopes and dreams of many climbers throughout history that made it, and more importantly representing the hopes and dreams of many more that couldn't make it. The climber touches the top, sits for a moment, looks at the Earth below and can know that they are now part of a league of people stretching back to Sir Edmund Hillary and Tenzing Norgay. But whilst they may have reached their dream and summitted, it is the journey home which is more important now.

*"It seemed difficult at first to grasp that we had got there. I was too tired and too conscious of the long way down to safety really, to feel any great elation. But as the fact of our success thrust itself more clearly into my mind, I felt a quiet glow of satisfaction spread through my body — a satisfaction less vociferous but more powerful than I had ever felt on a mountain top before"*. Words by Sir Edmund Hillary in his autobiography titled Our Ascent of the Everest.

As we have seen, through this climber's ascent, the process of aerobic respiration occurs when sufficient oxygen is delivered to cells and tissues. The rate of maximum oxygen uptake (something which we will revisit more in the chapter on marathon running) largely depends on the cardiac output, the ability to extract oxygen across the oxygen cascade and the mass of hemoglobin. The cardiac output at high altitude reaches a steady limit, partly to protect the heart muscle itself. In addition, the ability to extract oxygen does increase with minor physiological changes, but given the very small potential gradient possible confounded by lower pressures at high altitudes, this is again limited. Therefore, the only method left to enhance physical performance is to increase the oxygen content in the arterial system by enhancing the hemoglobin mass. To make the blood more concentrated, the kidneys continue to excrete fluid, thereby reducing the volume of blood in circulation while increasing the relative carrying capacity of blood. The kidneys also begin to secrete hormones into the body which increase the production of the donut-shaped red blood cells. One such hormone is called erythropoietin (EPO) and is particularly well known as many athletes abuse this in their attempts to gain a competitive advantage in physical performance.

At physiologically low $PaO_2$ around 40 mm Hg, EPO is released from the kidneys to increase hemoglobin transportation.

EPO is a glycoprotein hormone produced by cells called interstitial fibro-blasts in the kidney that signal for erythropoiesis (red blood cell production) in the bone marrow. It is nature's way of 'blood doping', where the number of red blood cells in the bloodstream is boosted in order to enhance athletic performance. Moreover, the number and penetration of fine blood vessels in the muscle tissue increases, bringing the cells closer and closer in proximity to the blood so that, once again as we saw in the lungs, the oxygen has the smallest possible distance to cross in order to reach the cells. This realm of science, perhaps driven by the commercial benefits of sporting success, has experienced a boom following the 1968 Olympics in Mexico City. At an altitude of 2,240 metres, it was speculated prior to these events how the higher altitude may impact the performances of these elite, world-class athletes, and most of the conclusions drawn were equivalent to those hypothesised. The endurance events suffered significantly, but the shorter sprint events were not substantially affected. These negative impacts were largely related to underperformance at high altitude while the beneficial effects in the latter group was attributed not only to less movement resistance due to the less dense air but also to the anaerobic nature of the sprint events. Ultimately, the games spawned an entire scientific discipline dedicated to utilising high altitude to facilitate athletic training and improve sporting performance, resulting in a variety of techniques such as 'Live High Train Low', 'Live High Train High', and 'Repeated Sprints in Hypoxia', and then artificially creating hypoxic conditions ranging from sleeping tents to entire hotels.

Over time, through the climb, the human body goes through a series of subtle changes which are all geared towards increasing the delivery of oxygen to tissue and the efficiency in which it is used in the body.

A physiology professor of mine during my degree programme, Professor Hugh Montgomery, has a great analogy to describe this effect. He used the example of a car embarking on a long drive with very little fuel. There are two options in this situation. The quicker and easier method is to get rid of all the excess weight in the vehicle so that less fuel is required per mile as the lower load reduces its work output. The second method, which is a more complex arrangement and takes longer to do, is to alter the engineering of the engine so that it actually burns fuel more efficiently. This second state is ultimately what the body tries to do!

At the centre of this process is the mitochondrial unit, in terms of both its presence and the way in which it works under this new stressful condition. We have already learnt how important this cellular organelle is in the production of energy in the body, and what we are beginning to discover is its plasticity. By that I mean the way in which its morphology, density and inner workings change under hypoxic, low oxygen conditions. Conducting incredibly painful muscle biopsies on one another's thighs while only a few hundred metres after descending from the summit of Mt. Everest and then again a few weeks later, a group of doctors were able to show that the number of mitochondrial units within our muscle fibres actually begins to decrease the longer we spend at high altitude. This process, although counterintuitive when we think about it, may actually occur in order to protect cells from the reduced oxygen concentration available. After all, in addition to producing the incredibly important ATP energy molecule in our body, mitochondria produces a number of highly reactive oxidative radicals which can have harmful effects on cells. Along with the reduction of mitochondria through alterations in the expression of genes responsible for mitochondria production, the units that are created also begin to alter the way in which they work and turn down the production of ATP molecules, again a system that appears designed to protect us at a cellular level. It is still however very early days in this journey and scientists are only beginning to scratch the surface of the real underlying process.

And it is this process which we are now beginning to unlock and discover as we strive to understand the true underlying mechanisms that allow the body to survive at high altitudes and with little oxygen. The 2019 Nobel Prize for Physiology or Medicine was awarded to three scientists working precisely in this field of study — how cells sense and adapt to oxygen availability and the discovery of the protein Hypoxic Inducible Factor (HIF), a transcription factor that regulates the oxygen-dependent responses seen in cells. The need for oxygen to sustain life has been understood since the onset of modern biology; but the molecular mechanisms underlying how cells adapt to variations in oxygen supply were unknown until the prize-winning work described by William Kaelin, Jr., Sir Peter Ratcliffe, and Gregg Semenza. With alterations in the fundamental biochemical pathways arising from the switching on and off of different genes, an environment is created within the cell in which its machinery is effectively able to become leaner and more efficient at utilising available oxygen. With time, these chronic changes that happen on a cellular level allow our body to perform magnificently complex feats, almost completely negating the fact that our body is under an incredibly harsh environment it was neither designed nor intended for. Summiting Mt. Everest is certainly one such feat!

# 2 The South Pole

*"I am just going outside and may be some time."*

**— Last words spoken by Lawrence Oates to
Captain Robert Falcon Scott, Terra Nova Expedition
to the South Pole 1912**

---

*Let us travel back in time to the wonderful city of London. It is June of
1910 and what a year it has been for Great Britain. There is a new King
on the throne, the mammoth 80,000 seater stadium of Old Trafford has
just been opened in Manchester and the English Channel has just been
crossed for the first time by a British-built plane. In addition to all these
great feats, one of the country's greatest explorers of all, Captain Robert
Falcon Scott, has his heart set on becoming the first man to reach the
icy bottom of the world, the South Pole. His ship, the Terra Nova, which
he bought for the princely sum of £12,500, was a whaling ship and had
seen plenty of action in the chilly Labrador Sea. Filled to the brim with
supplies, instruments, equipment and crew, the sturdy ship set sail on
the 15th of June from Cardiff. Making a stopover in Australia on his
way to the Antarctic continent, it was during this halt that Captain Scott
received a strange telegram from Captain Roald Amundsen, a celebrated
Norwegian explorer, which was about to turn his world upside down
forever. The words read, "Beg leave to inform you, Fram proceeding
Antarctic. Amundsen." And at this point in time, it suddenly dawned
on Scott that he was not alone in this great quest and desire for legacy.*

*He realised that this planned expedition, the British Antarctic Expedition, had just become a race against Amundsen's team 'Fram' to one of the most hostile and unforgiving landscapes on Earth.*

Setting sail today from the Southern Hemisphere, to reach its southernmost point — the South Pole, ships frequently land at Ross Island, an island formed by four volcanoes (including Mt. Erebus which is still active) in the Ross Sea near the continent of Antarctica. First claimed by New Zealand, because of the persistent presence of the ice sheet, the island is sometimes taken to be part of the Antarctic mainland. Ross Island was originally discovered in 1840 by Sir James Ross, and it was only later given its name (in honour of him) by Captain Robert Scott. Today Ross Island is home to New Zealand's Scott Base, and the largest Antarctic settlement, the U.S. Antarctic Program's McMurdo Station.

But let's travel back in time, well over a hundred years, to the famous race to the South Pole. Setting up camp on Ross Island Captain Scott had decided to follow the route that the infamous Polar explorer Ernest Shackleton had pioneered towards the Pole, up the Beardmore Glacier on to the Polar Plateau, in his 'Nimrod' Expedition of 1909 in which the Brit came within a hundred miles of the Pole but was forced to turn back due to bad weather. Finally, after many months of bunkering down in the snow and ice, on the 1st of November 1911, the race began and Scott left base camp with his team of support parties, motorised sledges, dogs and ponies for his long awaited journey south, which unfortunately for him was fated to be his last. On the 17th of Jan 1912, after three grueling months in the ice and snow, Scott and his team of five finally reached their goal. However, their celebrations were short-lived as they quickly discovered they were in fact too late as Amundsen's team had beaten them to it by 33 days. Awaiting them

at the Pole were the Norwegians' black marker flag as well as a
tent containing surplus equipment. Amundsen had even left Scott
a note to deliver to the King of Norway in case he did not return.
With a temperature of minus 30 degrees Celsius, the dispirited
men departed for home, but the ill effects of the cold and expedition living conditions had already taken a toll on their bodies and
their unfortunate downward spiral had begun. A few days after
Captain Oates, an expedition team member, was badly struck by
frostbite and was unable to go on, he courageously walked out of
his tent and was immortalised in history for his departing words, "I
am just going outside and may be some time." Captain Scott and
the remaining men lay in their sleeping bags confined to their tent
and gradually slipped away into a coma and finally death. In a cruel
twist of fate, the brave men were found only 11 miles away from
their supply depot. Scott's final diary entry read, *"We shall stick it
out to the end, but we are getting weaker, of course, and the end
cannot be far. It seems a pity but I do not think I can write more —
R Scott."* The race to the Pole was over. What led to the demise
of these brave souls will be the subject of this chapter, as we learn
how the frail human body is impacted by the negative temperatures and ice and wind. Our journey together will begin on the
Ross Ice Sheet itself, a point in which most expedition teams now
chose to begin their own polar journeys, and continue in the footsteps of these historic greats.

## McMurdo Sound

Our expedition team find themselves seated in a C17 aircraft; a
United States Air Force, military operated aeroplane. This win-
dowless cargo plane, devoid of any luxury, takes our team on a
5 hour flight from Christchurch, flying over southern island across the
ice sheet to land at McMurdo sound. A chilling outdoor temperature

of minus 25 degrees Celsius greets the team on landing. Arriving at McMurdo base, which is run by the United States government, whilst it is easy to think that a desolate environment would await them, the team is actually greeted to a collection of a hundred buildings, which can house 1200 residents and visitors in summer months.

French physiologist Claude Bernard wrote in 1878 that *"the milieu interieur never varies. All the vital mechanisms [...] have only one object, that of preserving constant the conditions of life in the internal environment."* The human body has a finely controlled temperature setting, the process and refinement of which happens completely outside of our conscious minds. Under normal conditions of health, this value is close to 37 degrees Celsius. This is not to say that our temperature is fixed at this value, but rather it represents the average value of its natural fluctuations throughout the day. The importance of this temperature control is that all the various functions of our cells occur through the actions of various enzymes made up of proteins, and these protein units function only within a tight temperature band. Too hot and they break up under a process called 'denaturation'; too cold and they simply freeze up and stop. How we landed on this particular functional temperature through the events of evolution is beyond the scope of this book (although some evidence suggests that this is a value which is warm enough to ward off infection — whilst maintaining an energy input that does not require us to be constantly eating all day to maintain the metabolic demands to generate this value), but what we do know is that mankind's dispersion across the planet has been largely driven by temperature and climate. Although we do find pockets of civilisation at some of the more extreme ends of the weather spectrum, by and large our species has flourished in less extreme and thus more habitable zones across Earth.

Before we get to the process of heat control known as thermoregulation, let us look at the way in which heat is managed between various objects. Heat transfer refers to the process whereby thermal energy is exchanged between various objects in space. This process can occur through four main methods, namely conduction, convection, radiation and evaporation, depending on the physical state of those objects (i.e., whether they are solids, liquids or gases). As stated in the second law of thermodynamics, heat energy, like all other types of energy in a natural state, flows from an area of high concentration to a lower one in order to try and reach a state of equilibrium. This is literally the microscopic exchange of energy from one vibrating atom to the next. When the body finds itself en route to the South Pole and having to brace itself against negative forty degree Celsius polar winds, the natural state for heat exchange is down its gradient and from the body to the outside environment. If left unchecked, as was the case for poor Captain Scott and his team, this can turn disastrous.

Shackleton's hut, on Ross Island, served as the expedition operations for the British 1907 Nimrod Expedition, an earlier attempt in the race to the geographic South Pole led by a young Ernest Shackleton. It was not Shackleton's first time on the Antarctic Ice Sheet, for he had been part of Robert Scott's Discovery Expedition but sent home, most likely suffering from scurvy. Originally his plan was to launch his own expedition from Scott's Discovery Hut, but was refused permission and therefore had to construct his own prefabricated hut at Cape Royds, just 23 miles from the original structure. The hut's simple 33 feet long by 19 feet wide structure was complete for the entire team, with separate lodging for the expedition's ponies, dogs, and the first motorcar on the continent, a 12-15 horsepower Arrol Johnston specially retrofitted for the expedition. Unfortunately for Shackleton and his crew, the expedition was plagued with challenges and his team was forced to turn back within 100 miles of the pole. The hut was restored in 2008 and to everyone's surprise the restoration team found five crates of whisky and brandy, intact and full, in 2006. Carefully removed from the ice four years later, one crate of whiskey has now been carefully exported to New Zealand, where conservators are attempting to slowly thaw the bottles. What a drink of history that would be!

In 2008, 100 years later a British team, led by the late Henry Worsley was formed of the direct descendents of Shackleton's original team, aimed to undertake the exact same journey made by their forefathers and this time reach the South Pole. They did so with success, exactly 100 years to the day later. In his diary records Henry recounted opening the door of the Shackleton Hut and the feelings that came over him of being there. From his book *In Shackleton's Footsteps* he wrote, *"There was too much to take in. The warmth of the place and its atmosphere was intriguing. It was easy to imagine being welcomed in by Shackelton and offered a tin mug of steaming tea. You could hear the chatter and the laughs (and the odd cough). You could smell the tobacco smoke, damp wool drying and coal burning in the stove. The past seemed vividly alive and it was easy to feel that this was still the home to untroubled spirits who had passed away in the dark and unforgiving months of the Antarctic Winter in 1908".*

So how does the body control its internal temperature, maintaining it to within a narrow band irrespective of external conditions? We begin first by looking at the way temperature is sensed. The body has two mechanisms for receiving information on its temperature. Located across the skin are microscopic nerve endings called peripheral thermoreceptors. Divided into two types — warm and cold — these nerve endings code absolute and relative changes in temperature and, depending on the change, the appropriate sensor fires a signal to the brain via a nerve. The higher the change in temperature, the faster the rate of firing and the stronger the impulse that is sent to the brain.

At this point I would like to spend a moment to discuss the mechanism by which peripheral nerve cells fire an electrical impulse and are thus able to communicate with the central nervous system comprising the spinal cord and brain. This mechanism is particularly important in the context of this chapter as we shall see later on when we examine the clinical implications of cold physiology and how certain tissue types can be manipulated to create a beneficial physiological effect.

Nerve cells, also known as neurons, are electrically excitable cells that receive, process, and transmit information through electrical or chemical signals and are made up of three distinct parts. The main command centre of the nerve cell is called the soma and this houses all the important functional units that control the activity of the cell. This is followed by a dendrite or axon, which are filamentous extensions of the cell, giving the nerve cell many fine connections which allow it to talk to other cells (the axon, which is the larger of the two, can sometimes be a metre or more in length!). Lastly, there is a space between two nerve cells which is called the synaptic junction. Nerve cells convey information to each other in the form of electrochemical impulses (known as nerve impulses or action potentials) carried by individual neurons that make up the nerve. These impulses are extremely fast, with some myelinated neurons conducting at speeds of up to 120 metres per second (myelin is a form of fat insulation that wraps itself around the axon of the nerve, helping it to conduct electrical impulses at a faster rate). The impulses then travel from one neuron to another by crossing the synaptic junction, the message being converted from an electrical one within the axon to a chemical one across the functional gap and then again back to an electrical one in the neighbouring neuron.

The amazing property of these spaces is that it is nothing like a normal, empty gap in the way we would imagine. The effect that is created at the postsynaptic neuron is determined not by the pre-synaptic neuron or chemical released as the neurotransmitter, but by the type of receptor that is activated on the other side of the cleft (sympatic space). We can think of neurotransmitters as being a key and the receptor as a lock; the only difference in this key metaphor is that the same type of key can be used to open many different types of locks. Overall, receptors can be classified either as *excitatory* (causing an increase in firing rate), *inhibitory* (causing a decrease in firing rate), or *modulatory* (causing long-lasting effects not directly related to firing rate). Therefore, the purpose of the synaptic junction is to allow nerve fibres from different regions to converge and 'talk' to one another. This conversation can be exaggerated or dampened according to the needs of the organism at that point in time. The arrival of the nerve impulse at the junction triggers the opening of voltage-gated calcium channels at the end membrane in order for the nerve impulse to enter the terminal. In turn, this causes the microscopic chemical-filled vesicles to fuse with the terminal membrane and release the neurotransmitter into the cleft. The neurotransmitters then diffuse across the synaptic cleft, activate receptors on the postsynaptic neuron, and propagate the nerve impulse to the adjacent neuron.

The two most prevalent neurotransmitter chemicals in the central nervous system, particularly the brain, are glutamate and gamma-aminobutyric acid (GABA). Glutamate acts on several types of receptors and have both excitatory and modulatory effects. GABA, on the other hand, acts on different receptors, all of which are inhibitory. It is estimated that each of the one hundred billion neurons in our brains has on average 7,000 synaptic connections to other neurons. Data suggests that the brain of a three year-old child has about one quadrillion synapses which, while declining with age, stabilise at around 100 to 500 trillion synapses by adulthood!

Action potential refers to the process of electrical messaging within a nerve cell. An action potential is a very short event in which the electrical membrane potential of a cell rises and then rapidly falls again sequentially along the length of an axon, therefore passing a message from the neuron to the synaptic junction. Action potentials in themselves are merely a message being transduced and they have different effects depending on the final cell it is in contact with. For example, action potentials in the heart's cardiac myocyte cells lead to rhythmical contractions, whereas action potentials within the pancreas gland lead to the secretion of insulin by its beta cells. The body has amazingly created one underlying methodology that different types of cells can use for their own unique ends. Luckily for us the science is essentially the same and therefore worthwhile considering in the context of this topic.

Ordinarily, as we have seen, the human body and nature tends to favour a state of equilibrium. Any deviation away from equilibrium requires energy and therefore work must be done! Our nerve cells have found a way to manipulate this need for equilibrium in order to make the transmission of impulses more efficient. Situated along the length of an axon are tiny microscopic pumps and channels that allow the movement of two very important charged atoms, sodium which is denoted by $Na^+$ and potassium which is denoted by $K^+$ At rest, the neuron begins by actively pumping $K^+$ ions (the charged version of a potassium atom) out of the cell across its membrane through these little $K^+$ pumps. As this is an active process that goes against the natural equilibrium state, it requires ATP molecules which, as we have seen in Chapter 1, are the energy currency of our cells. As more and more positively charged potassium ions are moved to the outside milieu, the inside of the cell becomes relatively negative. This state of relative electrical difference creates the 'resting potential' wherein the nerve is now charged and ready to kick into action when called up. Once the neuron receives the signal to transduce, it opens the protein channels embedded within its membrane which then allows $Na^+$ ions to enter. Remembering that the inside of the membrane is now negative versus the outside, these positively charged $Na^+$ ions flow down its electrical gradient and enters the cell. This changes the electrochemical gradient within the nerve cell, which in turn produces a further rise in the membrane potential and makes it increasingly positive. This then causes more channels to open, producing a greater electric current across the cell membrane, and so on. The process proceeds explosively until all available ion channels are open, resulting in a large upswing in the membrane potential. Thus, an action potential is created which makes its way along the entire length of the neuron, thereby allowing a message to be carried through the body.

Thinner neurons and axons require less metabolic expense to produce and carry action potentials than thicker ones, but the thicker axons convey impulses more rapidly. Therefore, to minimize the metabolic expense while still maintaining rapid conduction, many neurons insulate themselves with a fatty sheath of myelin wrapped around their axons. Exquisite physiology doesn't stop there though, for neurons have an additional trick up their metaphorical sleeves to quicken the process further. The sheathes themselves are not one continuous covering of myelin but are instead grouped in bands that expose unmyelinated regions of the axonal membrane at regular intervals. It is at these unexposed regions, called nodes of Ranvier, where membrane equilibrium activity can occur, resulting in action potentials effectively 'jumping' from one node to the next rather than having to be transmitted down the entire length of the axon. This saltatory conduction (from the latin word *saltare* meaning to jump) allows for conduction speeds close to 150 metres per second instead of 10 metres per second, which it would have otherwise been if the entire length of the axon had to undergo a change in its membrane potential. The very last adaptation of these nerve units is the principle of 'all or nothing' where the impulse must be fired to the extent that the threshold for generating an action potential is reached. Any smaller stimuli that begins to activate some voltage-gated Na pumps but fails to reach the threshold does not transmit a message. Likewise, a stronger stimulus does not produce a stronger signal but instead increases the frequency of nerve firing, translating into the brain interpreting this input as being a stronger message to act upon.

Now that we are aware of the elegance of the process in which messages such as being cold are transmitted through the body, let us return to the peripheral temperature sensors in our body which are continuously helping us to monitor the environment. But just before we do, lets return to our expedition team, who's brave efforts over the past ten days have taken them to the Ross Ice Shelf.

## Ross Ice Shelf

It may be larger than the area of France, it may be several hundred metres thick, and it may have a near vertical 50 metre high ice face that stretches almost 600 kilometres across; but the most fascinating part of the Ross Ice Shelf is that 90% of it is actually underwater! Discovered in 1841 by James Ross, the British Commander spent two years trying to find an open water path through it to the South Pole but finally concluded *"Well, there's no more chance of sailing through that than through the cliffs of Dover"*. From then on, the Ross Ice Shelf represents the first phase of a Polar expedition. The shelf is fed primarily by giant glaciers, or ice streams, that transport ice down to it from the high polar ice sheet of East and West Antarctica. Thus, although the barrier's position appears almost stationary, it actually undergoes continual change by calving and melting that accompany northward movement of the shelf ice. It can be a chilling minus forty degrees celsius on most days; and its a good thing that our bodies have a variety of ways to keep track of the environment around it.

There are two types of peripheral sensors. One is set in our skin and covers our entire body; the others are located around our main organs and relay messages back to the brain about the internal temperature states of our big tissues. These peripheral signals are modulated along with inputs that feed in from the central thermoreceptors which are located within the brain and the spinal cord. These centralised receptors measure the temperature of the blood flowing through and feed millions of bytes of information to a tiny primordial part of the brain called the hypothalamus, buried deep within the brain tissue just above the brainstem.

The hypothalamus is roughly the size of a pea and weighs about 1% of the entire weight of the brain. Yet, as shown time and time again in human physiology, size does not matter and this little organ is one of the most highly connected parts of the brain and is responsible for many important autonomic brain functions. As well as being a sensory command centre within the body, it also has an output capability and secretes many hormones into the bloodstream that serve a wide variety of functions ranging from temperature control to growth, reproduction, sleep, stress, urine output and much more! Warmth receptors are composed of unmyelinated C-fibres with slow conduction velocities, whereas those responding to the cold are made up of these C-fibres as well as larger myelinated A-delta fibres that conduct at much higher speeds. Notably, there is a paradoxical response whereby cold fibres fire action potentials to very high temperatures (above 45 degrees Celsius), the reason for which is not understood.

The first time I experienced conditions anywhere near what Captain Scott did when he first reached the Ross ice sheet was on an expedition to the Arctic Circle in Siberia. One of the objectives of this visit was to measure and analyse the body's response to environmental stress, such as the Arctic conditions and temperatures well below minus ten degrees Celsius. Also called the Yamal-Nenets region, which translates to 'edge of the world', temperatures in this part of the Earth on the outskirts of Russia often drop to minus 50 degrees Celsius. Amazingly, even in this isolated and extreme landscape, human beings exist (and thrive). A small nomadic tribe known as the Nenets live in reindeer-hide teepees, dress in reindeer-hide fur clothes, eat raw reindeer meat, sacrifice animals to the gods of their ancient religion and migrate more than 1,000 miles each year on hand-made, wooden sledges. Around 10,000 strong, the tribe commands a reindeer flock of almost 300,000. These families follow the natural migration patterns of the reindeer, travelling across the flat, bleak terrain and the frozen waters of the Ob River. Amongst all the various experimentations and physical activities we did during our trip, one of the most striking moments for me occurred after a return from a summit climb on one of the mountains in the region. The locals had caught and killed a reindeer right in front of our group, after which they stripped it of its flesh and fur and dissected most of its internal organs, showing us how they used almost every single part of this majestic creature which they rely upon so dearly. A local tribesman then took a cup and reached down into the freshly opened abdomen of the beast, scooping up a cup full of blood and offering it to me as a sign of friendship. I felt very obliged to accept the offer! This is a memory that will stay with me always.

## Beardmore Glacier

As our brave expedition team nears its half way mark, it meets the next key obstacle along its polar expedition. Descending almost 2500 metres from the Ross Ice Shelf, at 200 km long and 40 km wide the Beardmore Glacier is one of the largest in the world.

The glacier is one of the main passages through the Transantarctic Mountains to the great polar plateau beyond, and was one of the early routes to the South Pole despite its steep upward incline. Shackleton is likely to have been the first human to ever set foot upon it and named it after Sir William Beardmore, a Scottish industrialist and the sponsor of his 1908 Nimrod Expedition.

A few years later, it was Captain Scott and his party to the South Pole in 1911 who were the first people to collect rock samples from the Transantarctic Mountains in the Beardmore Glacier region. Some of which contained fossilised plants which suggested that in the distant geological past Antarctica had a tropical climate. These findings helped contribute to the hypothesis, which was contested at the time, for plate tectonics and the movement of the Earth's crust.

Descending on to it from The Gateway, the hard blue glacier ice is covered with a light layer of snow. Weary expedition team members quickly rope themselves up as they recognize the tell tale shadows and cracks on its surface of the hundreds of small crevasses that lie in their path, not huge gaping chasms but narrow slits, well camouflaged by the fallen snow but large enough to fall in and break a leg or twist a knee — especially if travelling on only boots and crampons.

The ice of course has its advantages, as sleds move more freely over it, friction free, but will take on a mind of its own as it bumps and crashes along behind. A team's speed will thus ultimately be dictated by the amount of twisted and rubblised ice that they have to negotiate on their route up the glacier. The lack of fresh ample snow also means longer melting times at night to create fresh water, and water which then also contains fine silt and moraine. But all of this makes for breathtaking scenery, as the glacier weaves its way through the mountains and the blues and white reflect the clear bright sun. Climbing up in the gentle incline finally reaches its toughest point, just before its exit, as the gradient steepens making the sleds pull heavily on the expedition team's backs. Successfully climbing it, the glacier's exit point is marked by a three peaked feature called Buckley Island. It's a tough few weeks and the team's battered and bruised bodies are now beginning to feel the wear and tear being put upon it and the harsh realities of this physical, and increasing mental, journey.

Part of the responses we shall now look at in more detail are the events that play out from the activation of the 'antidrop' centre located in the posterior portion of the hypothalamic thermostat. When faced with a fall in ambient and thus bodily temperature, the body activates two main mechanisms — one reduces the loss of heat from the body and the other increases the internal generation of heat. One small point to note is that in addition to our involuntary physiological mechanisms (which we will also examine in this chapter), there are also voluntary actions that occur through the involvement of the higher brain known as the cerebral cortex. These include things like wearing warmer clothes, preferring warmer habitats, eating food and promoting warmth by walking around or huddling up. However, this book aims to highlight some of the very elegant physiological responses that occur in the human body when life is pushed to the limits of survival and thus I will be focusing more on our involuntary responses for the remainder of this chapter.

As we begin to look at this process in greater detail, it makes sense to remind ourselves of what we notice when we are exposed to the cold. One of the very first things we have all probably observed is that we get goosebumps all over and our skin begins to turn pale. Why does this happen and why is this reaction to the cold so similar to when we are scared (the phrase *"you look like you have just seen a ghost!"* comes to mind)? The answer partly lies in the autonomic nervous system; that is, the part that is not under conscious control, which we call the sympathetic system. Scientists call this part of the autonomic nervous system the 'fight or flight' centre and it evolved to allow us to respond quickly to dangerous or threatening situations, such as running away from a sabre-toothed tiger during the ice age! This system activates a series of events in the body primarily through the secretion of stress hormones into the bloodstream. These protein messengers travel via the bloodstream to various target organs and bring about the changes we need to help the body defend itself or flee from a dangerous situation. Being stranded on the Antarctic Plateau or waiting for the bus on a winter's morning elicits the same response.

As the sympathetic nervous system kicks into action, the first thing we notice is that the tiny hairs that cover our bodies begin to stand. Microscopic piloerector muscles that inhabit our skin cells contract, calling the hair cells to attention and creating an envelope of air around our body that reduces heat loss through air conduction. Additionally, the activity of these nerves in our blood vessels release the hormone noradrenaline, causing the constriction of small capillaries located under our skin. This vasoconstriction reduces blood flow to the peripheries of our body, thereby reducing heat loss via convection to the external atmosphere. The redirection of blood also supplies warm blood to core organs like the brain, heart, gut and kidneys and maintains the normal conditions required to keep us alive. One more main effect of the sympathetic nervous system is the release of another hormone called adrenaline into the bloodstream via the adrenal cortex located above the kidneys. Adrenaline has many effects on the body and we shall learn more about them in later chapters, but for the purposes of surviving in the cold, its main effect is to increase the generation of heat in the body by raising our basal metabolic rate.

With heat generation through hormonal control, the hypo-thalamus also controls the secretion of thyroid hormones from the thyroid gland. Similar to adrenaline, these hormones increase the body's basal metabolic rate and generate heat to the core organs. The last main effect of the heat generation system is the phenom-enon of shivering. Something which we have all experienced at some point in our lives, shivering is a process that, although seem-ingly crude, is in fact a very elegant mechanism for producing heat throughout the body.

Located deep within the posterior of the hypothalamus is an area called the primary motor centre for shivering. This area is normally inhibited by signals from the heat centre and excited by cold signals that are generated from the skin and spinal cord. Therefore, this centre becomes activated when body temperature falls even a fraction below our preset critical temperature level. The shivering reflex is then triggered, which coordinates a series of rhythmic contractions in the skeletal muscle across our body. The byproduct of this utilisation of energy is the production of heat. Although seemingly useful in response to cold, this process is however a double-edged sword because the contraction of mus-cles requires a supply of blood. As we already saw earlier in this chapter, the sympathetic activity in the body results in vasocon-striction in an attempt to reduce blood flow to the skin and prevent heat loss. However, the longer we shiver, the greater the muscles' requirement for blood, resulting in a paradox that the body must deal with — to supply blood to enable shivering while losing heat through convection. Moreover, the shivering reflex activates skele-tal muscle across our body. At small temperature drops, these con-tractions are insignificant and do not bother us. However, as the temperature continues to fall and the shivering reflex gets stron-ger and stronger, whole limbs can become ineffective and this can be severely disadvantageous to the organism on the whole. If you have ever found yourself trying to swim after plunging into an ice-cold pool, you will understand what I mean. The contractions that affect our arms and legs can render useful movement almost impossible and this is thought to be one of the main reasons why so many people drown when they drop through an ice sheet into the freezing water below — they are simply unable to swim in a coordinated and effective manner.

One last elegant adaptation our bodies have, something which we share with many animals and particularly those that hibernate, is brown fat. Like the name suggests, it is a type of adipose tissue, but unlike the harmful white version that fills our bellies and clogs our arteries, this version is useful for heat generation and maintenance. Brown adipocytes (fat cells) contain numerous small droplets of fat and a much higher number of iron-containing mitochondria, which gives brown adipocytes their distinctive color. These smaller fat droplets are easier to 'burn' in order for mitochondria to create energy and therefore heat. It was once thought that only newborns and infants had these cells as they have little or no shivering response and that we lose this material as we grow older. However, recent studies on adults show that specifically those individuals who spend a lot of time in colder climates retain this version of fatty cells, reflecting their bodies' attempt to adapt to the harsh environment.

The southernmost continent of Antarctica — the unforgiving mass of wind, snow and ice and arguably one of Earth's most formidable landscapes — is so cold that its temperature in winter is sometimes almost the same as the temperature on Mars. With an ice sheet that is almost two miles thick, Antarctica is the windiest, coldest, driest and highest continent on the planet. As we have seen through this chapter, mankind's innate ambition for conquest has led many to try to reach the South Pole, and many have failed in their valiant attempts. But these problems are not just restricted to the adventurous few; any inhabitants trying to cope with a bad winter will have an appreciation of the difficulties associated with dealing with extreme cold. A mild injury that afflicts many is the condition called chilblain. This condition is a consequence of the cold weather in combination with moisture or humidity. The cold exposure damages capillary beds in the skin typically in the limbs, which in turn causes redness, itching, blisters, and inflammation. Although usually nothing more serious than a temporary inconvenience, frostnip and frostbite can quickly follow.

While frostnip refers to the superficial version of the damage spectrum which does not destroy cells, frostbite occurs when there is localised damage to the skin's deeper tissues. We have already seen that under conditions of intense cold, the body induces a systemic constrictor response on blood vessels in the periphery in its protective response to conserve core body warmth. Over prolonged periods of time, however, this protective response can have disastrous and often irreversible effects on the tissues and blood vessels. Chapter 1 illustrated the importance of oxygen delivery to our tissues which happens through the blood vessel network. As blood gets cut off from tissue, the buildup of toxins, lack of oxygen and lack of fuels to produce energy gradually lead to cellular death, something we call necrosis.

This destructive process begins with a superficial injury which is called either 'stage one' or frostnip. In this condition, the skin freezes and the person experiences pain and itching. The skin changes colour and develops patches of red, yellow and white areas that become numb. If treated early, this stage of the disease is reversible with minimal long-term damage. If the cold continues, the skin begins to freeze and the person develops blisters that blacken and harden. This level two injury often appears worse than it really is and healing typically occurs within a month albeit with some long-term damage, mainly an insensitivity to heat and cold. If the area freezes further, deep frostbite will occur. This stage three and four injury results in muscles, tendons, blood vessels and nerves freezing permanently. The skin becomes hard and the use of the area is lost. The deep frostbite results in bloodfilled purplish and black blisters that, ironically due to the underlying nerve damage in the area, are often painless. This extreme form of frostbite may result in fingers and toes being amputated (at times dropping off on their own!) and can more seriously become infected with gangrene, which can lead to sepsis and death. And while these conditions are painful, inconvenient and physically disturbing, chiefly to blame in the many thousands of deaths that have occurred due to cold is our susceptibility to hypothermia.

*"The blood had left the surface of his body and he now began to shake from the cold. Even with the strong effort that he made, his trembling fingers would not obey and the sticks were hopelessly scattered.... the man looked down at his hands to locate them and found them hanging on the ends of his arms. He thought it curious that it was necessary to use his eyes to discover where his hands were.*

*He began waving his arms, beating the mittened hands against his sides. He did this for five minutes. His heart produced enough blood to stop his shaking. But no feeling was created in his hands. He did not shake any more.*

*As he sat and regained his breath, he noted that he was feeling warm and comfortable. He was not shaking, and it even seemed that a warm glow had come to his body. And yet, when he touched his nose or face, there was no feeling..... It was his last moment of fear. When he had recovered his breath and his control, he sat and thought about meeting death with dignity.*

*With this newfound peace of mind came the first sleepiness. A good idea, he thought, to sleep his way to death. Freezing was not as bad as people thought. There were many worse ways to die."* These words are from Jack London's famous short story, *To Build a Fire*, written in 1908 and which beautifully describes the range of emotions the unnamed main character went through as he faced the inevitability of death along the Yukon trail in Canada.

Hypothermia is the condition in which the body's core temperature drops below 35 degrees Celsius, the temperature needed for the many thousands of normal protein interactions and metabolic processes of our cells. The symptoms associated with the milder form of the disease are often vague, but when we recall our worst days out on the ski slopes or being trapped by bad weather trekking in the hills, most of us have probably suffered from this condition at some point during our thrill seeking, adventurous moments! As the temperature falls, our sympathetic nervous system kicks in and the body triggers the shivering reflex and peripheral vasoconstriction. Internally the rise in stress hormones raises our heart rate, blood pressure and ventilation rate in an attempt to increase oxygenation in cold tissues. These hormones also send messages to the liver to increase the production of glucose from our reserves, again in an attempt to manage the freezing tissues.

As the temperature drops further, the shivering mechanism becomes more violent and uncoordinated and useful movement becomes a struggle (*note the character's inability to strike a match to light a fire*). Although subjects appear alert, confusion sets in and this affects our ability to make rational decisions, thereby contributing to potentially fatal outcomes. Many climbers anecdotally remember the strange decisions they made, often in very precipitous moments on a climb, only realising later that these are often the result of hypothermia causing them to be unable to think straight. As the body attempts to conserve more heat, the arms, legs, hands and face shut down even more and a blue hue sets in.

Below 28 degrees Celsius, severe hypothermia ensues and now the normal physiological responses of the body no longer function. Paradoxically, the heart and breathing rate and the blood pressure all begin to decrease and most cellular processes begin to shut down (*the character noticed that his breathing slowed*). The subject is often unable to perform any meaningful motor activity and experiences a very drowsy and near comatose mental state. This triggers two very primordial reflexes which are hidden deep in our subconscious and are remnants of our evolutionary past. The first is terminal burrowing, which is a self-protective mechanism and what many call the 'hide and die' syndrome. The individual looks to enter a small, enclosed space and researchers claim that this is an autonomous process of the brain stem triggered in the final state of hypothermia, producing a primitive burrowing-like behavior as seen in hibernating animals. The other response is paradoxical undressing and happens when the combative and severely confused subject begins to shed their clothes. One explanation for this effect is a cold-induced malfunction of the hypothalamus, which is now no longer able to correctly sense the correct body temperature. The other explanation is that the vascular smooth muscles which contract in order to reduce heat loss become exhausted (known as a loss of vasomotor tone) and begin to relax, leading to a sudden surge of blood and heat to the extremities, thereby fooling the person into feeling overheated (*our character felt a sudden warm glow flow through his body just before he slipped off in a deep sleep*). This rather peaceful description of hypothermia, something which we can easily imagine happened to the Scott's crew at the beginning of the chapter, is in stark contrast to the events that occur when a person falls into icy waters. If prolonged, this too can lead to a drop in the body's core temperature, but the reaction is often more violent and worth exploring in more detail.

Walking across an ice sheet on a frozen lake is perhaps one of the most heart-racing things one can do, for the mild adventurer that is! The apprehension of falling through and the worry of survival all contribute to the excitement. Fortunately, I have never encountered the cold shock response, the physiological event that occurs when one finds oneself unlucky enough to have fallen through. On encountering the freezing temperature, the human body undergoes an automated gasp reflex in response to the sudden skin cooling. This can be fatal when the person is underwater and is therefore one of the key reasons a life jacket is recommended irrespective of a person's ability to swim. This reflex is then followed by an increase in the breathing rate. This hyperventilation begins as a response to the cold but can be exacerbated as the person becomes increasingly anxious and afraid. The rapid breathing reduces the levels of carbon dioxide in the blood and can cause drowsiness and confusion. Thus, it is vitally important to try and remain calm and to concentrate and take control of one's breathing should this happen. As time goes by and the subject remains in the cold water, the constricted peripheral blood flow makes the heart work harder and harder for the blood to keep circulating and supply oxygen to our muscles so that we can continue swimming. For people who have underlying cardiac problems or diseases in their coronary vessels, this can precipitate a cardiac arrest. Finally, the body succumbs to hypothermia as it continues to lose heat to the water, an effect which occurs at a faster rate than heat loss to air.

*The year is 2060. The crew of the Explorer are at the apogee of its orbit around Earth and are preparing to fire its deep space engine in its journey to Titan, one of the moons of Saturn. Having successfully landed on Mars in 2032, mankind's taste for space exploration has intensified and the human race has set itself an ambitious course to explore more of our solar system for signs of life and future habitation. The International Space Exploration Agency, a collection of national-level agencies, has assembled a team of five scientists and researchers to brave the journey. With a 13-year round journey, the crew will spend the vast majority of its six-year outbound journey in a state of cryohibernation in order to preserve fuel and resources for its eight months-long study of the satellite's surface. The onboard doctor has examined the crew and inserted a dual bore cannula in the astronauts' brachial vein. The device called the umbilicus connects the individual to the cryostat life support device and, on entering the radiation-protected capsule, the crew gently slips off into a long slumber as the infusion matrix makes its way into each individual and takes over a number of physiological systems in order to render a state of prolonged hibernation.*

You may wonder what the above paragraph has got to do with my earlier writing on survival at the South Pole. Why I have suddenly veered off popular science and begun entering the realms of science fiction? Fiction it may be, but the content is rooted in scientific research and reflects a strong possibility of what lies ahead for mankind and the future of space travel. Early on in my description of the different physiological changes under cold conditions, I remarked that there are indeed practical benefits from having a better understanding of these adaptations, in particular to exploit the underlying mechanisms to our benefit.

Cryotherapy, the term used to describe the process of exploiting cold physiology already has a number of uses in medical science. From the simple use of ice packs during sports injuries, which help to reduce inflammation and pain in swollen joints or torn muscle, to the use of cryotherapy sprays to remove warts and moles, such therapies based on cold physiology are slowly beginning to play a larger and more significant role in medicine. But the really interesting applications — the stuff of science fiction — are already entering into the realms of everyday science and can potentially transform the way we treat diseases like cardiac arrests and strokes as well as facilitate mankind's quest to explore science more deeply, and maybe even live forever.

As we learned earlier in this chapter, at a very basic level, a reduction in tissue temperature can have a profound effect on the transmission of nerve impulses. Being proteins, the activity of the sodium and potassium channels that create the resting membrane potential can be inhibited, including the electrical impulses that carry the message of pain. This has important implications for individuals suffering from a cardiac arrest. Heart attacks occur when there is a disruption of blood flow to the heart which stops the pumping action needed to push blood around the body. As blood flow stops, these tissues are deprived of oxygen (we learnt how important this was in Chapter 1) while the buildup of toxins reaches dire levels. One way to reduce the cells' requirement for fuel and prevent toxin buildup during this acute event is to therapeutically induce hypothermia in the patient, reducing their core temperature to 33 degrees Celsius. This can be done in a variety of ways such as cold drips, cooling pads or cooling catheters.

In contrast to the accidental hypothermia we suffer from falling into a frozen lake, therapeutic mild hypothermia is administered in a controlled manner and it is believed to work in multiple ways. The return of blood flow to the brain and tissues after successful resuscitation, although essential and effective in restoring energy stores, can also trigger the release of harmful chemicals like free radicals, glutamate and other hormones, thus leading to multiple areas of cell death in the vital organs. By cooling the tissues, we effectively reduce their requirement for fuels as well as their ability to create these harmful substances. Doctors are beginning to utilise this physiological response in resuscitation rooms and operating theatres around the world.

The Kjølen mountain range is a series of steep, jagged and icy peaks that lie between Sweden and Norway. Set deeply away from any major forms of civilisation, the miraculous survival story of medical student Anna Bågenholm in 1999 changed our understanding of the boundaries between life and death forever. While skiing off-piste, Anna lost her footing and crashed through a frozen river where she was trapped under more than 6 inches of ice. After an hour of struggling, Anna's heart stopped beating and she laid dead, or at least that's what everyone thought. Her body was recovered and she was taken to the nearest hospital 100 miles away where her body temperature was measured as 13.7 degrees Celsius and she was assumed to be as dead as can be. Fortunately for her, Dr. Mads Gilbert was heading the emergency room that day and he believed that *"you're only dead if you're warm and dead!"* He knew that while lowering the body temperature will stop the heart, it also reduces tissue demand for oxygen and most importantly those of the brain cells. He later said in an interview, *"On the one side it can protect you but, on the other side, it will kill you. But it's all a question of how controlled the hypothermia is. Anna was probably cooled quite slowly but efficiently so that, when her heart stopped, her brain was already so cold that the oxygen need in the brain cells was down to zero... buying emergency services an extra time window to try and save the person's life."*

Measuring her blood's plasma potassium levels revealed near normal values, an indicator that the cell damage was minimal, and prompted Dr. Gilbert's decision to slowly warm Anna up. Four and a half hours after she fell through the ice, Anna's heart was successfully restarted. Amazingly, she spent the next 35 days on a life support machine in intensive care before being moved to a rehabilitation unit. From there, she began the slow process of training and restoring herself back to complete functioning. Anna is now Dr. Bågenholm and is a radiology consultant in the same hospital where her life was saved. She remains the coldest ever recorded human being to have lived to tell her story of near tragedy. To this day, she continues to ski in the mountains of northern Norway, a living reminder of the human body's incredible capacity for endurance and survival.

## The South Pole

I wonder how many people have dreamed of making it to the South Pole? What images conjure up as we think about what it must be like to reach it? A desolate, un-inhabited, extra-terrestrial like landscape, completely devoid of human life and activity? Well, unfortunately this isn't the case. Since the establishment of the United States Amundsen–Scott South Pole Station in 1956, there are now human beings living and working at the South Pole all year round.

The latest construction, which was opened in 2008, is an 80,000 square foot facility, costing roughly USD 150 million dollars and built to accommodate around 200 researchers. Since this station is at the only inhabited place on the land surface of the Earth from which the Sun is continuously visible for six months and is then continuously dark for the next six months; during each year, this station effectively experiences one extremely long 'day' and one equally long 'night'. And during this six-month 'night', the air temperatures can drop so low as to become minus 70 degrees celsius.

This station lies around 100 metres away from the true Geographic South Pole (our planet also has a magnetic South Pole, which is a different location), and because this station is located on a moving glacier, this station is actually being carried towards the South Pole, roughly at a rate of about 10 metres per year!

A person reaching the South Pole, after days if not weeks of isolated walking, is suddenly greeted by a flurry of human activity. What greets the person at the actual point of 'furthest south' (i.e. 90 degree south) is a tall grey rod, a plaque marking the historic race between Amundsen and Scott and a large american flag. The real photo opportunity is actually a few hundred metres away where there is a shorter red and white pole, atop which sits a brightly polished steel-silver orb, and surrounded by the flags of all the international partners that conduct research on the continent of Antarctica. Then walking inside the permanently staffed building, an expedition team member can buy a souvenir from its quintessential gift shop or eat at its fast food serving canteen. It seems consumer society really can reach any point on this planet!

And so a race which began more than a hundred years ago kickstarted a scientific journey to understand and ultimately exploit the physiological changes that our tissues undergo when they are challenged by cold environments. From the desolate Antarctic desert in the last century to the possibility of reaching out to new worlds in the next, we will continue studying the cold in order to push life further along its edge.

# Chapter 3 Marathons

"We have won!" Thersipus of Erchius exclaimed before collapsing and dying as he reached the city of Athens following the battle of Marathon.

— The Legend of Pheidippides, 490 B.C.

---

It felt as though a spring had suddenly snapped. Out of the blue I had the most excruciating pain on the outside of my right knee, like nothing I had experienced before. I was still 8 kilometres away from the finish line and I realised that this moment was when the real test would begin. It was my first ever marathon and I was desperate to do well. I had trained religiously over the last four months, sacrificing so much of life just to get to the start line. It's all too easy to give up, to convince ourselves that we are not ready or be overcome by the fear of failure and embarrassment. But that wasn't me. I have always tried to step outside my comfort zone and do things that are physically and mentally difficult. That's where real strength comes from, and I knew that this is what I needed to muster from deep within myself if I was going to have a chance at completing this race today. My knee was taped up for a pre-existing muscle injury and there wasn't any obvious swelling that I could see. I stopped at the medical tent to ice it and spray my leg with cold topical pain relief and then I continued on. It was probably the slowest I had ever run, taking me almost an hour and a half to reach the finish line from that point.

*Each stride was like a dagger to the knee, each pounding step a tear in my thigh. It was the spirit of the crowd that kept me going — familiar faces of friends along the route encouraging me on, some who actually ran alongside me for short stretches and complete strangers who just came to watch and cheer. As I reached the finish line, I had welled up with tears. How much of it was the physical pain I was enduring and how much was from the overpowering sense of achievement, I cannot tell. But I had done it and the best part was that I wasn't alone. Somewhere amongst the thousands of finishers was my wife and I was dead proud to have shared this journey of achievement with her too!*

— Personal Account of my first Marathon event

42.195 kilometres. 26 miles and 385 yards. The average runner takes around 50,000 strides to complete the race of all races — the marathon. Men and women have, for hundreds of years, raced one another along this seemingly arbitrary distance and for what, prizes and glory? Unfortunately no. Whilst only the most elite runners do gain financially from winning, if you ask most participants why they run, you are almost certainly going to hear that it is for the satisfaction gained in completing the marathon, pushing our body to its physical limit and accomplishing what many regard as a seemingly impossible physiological endeavour. This chapter embarks on a journey along the route of one of the newest and most exciting marathons in the world, the Mumbai Marathon. And as we join our runners along this route, I aim to walk (or rather run!) through the physiological changes in the human body as it completes one of the most physically demanding challenges ever created by mankind.

First run as part of the modern Olympic Games movement in 1896, the name 'marathon' originates from the legend of Pheidippides, a Greek messenger, around 490 B.C. As a professional running courier, Pheidippides (or Thersipus as he was known in other accounts) was tasked to take messages from one part of the Greek empire to another in a time long before any form of electronic communication existed. Humans were used instead of horses as they were able to cover much longer distances without tiring. Legend states that Pheidippides was sent from the battle-field of Marathon to Athens to announce that the Persians had been defeated. Running the distance of approximately 41 km non-stop, he burst into the courts to exclaim '*chairete, nikomen*' or '*Hail, we are the winners!*' only to then collapse and die. Although schol-ars throughout history have argued about the factual accuracy of this event, what the actual distance was, who the lone messenger really was and even whether the event ever happened, humanity has romanticised this legend and honoured it by establishing the event called the marathon.

The first official version of the race was won, quite aptly, by a Greek man named Spyridon 'Spyros' Louis, who was a water car-rier by profession, and he took 2 hours 58 minutes and 50 seconds to complete. It was not until the 1984 Summer Olympics in Los Angeles that women were allowed to compete in the race. Today, the world record for the fastest completion stands at 2:01:39, set at the 2018 Berlin Marathon by Eliud Kipchoge, making it his third win at Berlin and the first time in history that the run was com-pleted under 2:02, a time that many thought was impossible to beat. A record which, since the writing of this chapter, has been beaten by the very same runner in a controlled event held in Vienna. This is the first time in history in which a human being has run a marathon distance race in under 2 hours (refer to Chapter 8, on 'Mind Over Matter' for more details). Annually there are almost 500 official marathons that are organised across more than 80 countries. There is also an ever increasing list of variations including The Midnight

Sun Marathon in Norway, the South Africa Big 5 Marathon through safari parks, the Great Wall run in China and the Everest Marathon from Naamche Bazaar to Lukla.

So just how stressful is running a marathon to the human body? Considering the physical endurance needed to pump out 50,000-odd strides to completion, the more than 15-fold increase in metabolic rate, and the heavy workload strain on the heart and cardiovascular system, most people, when asked, believe that running a marathon is too extreme to be associated with healthy living. While this may be the sentiment today, even as recent as the late 1970s, many scientists and doctors believed that marathon running actually afforded lifelong immunity against the deposition of dangerous fatty plaques along our coronary blood vessels, thus conferring protection to runners from cardiovascular diseases. This theory was however finally overturned in a very unfortunate case report of Jim Fixx in 1987. Jim was an overweight, overstressed smoker whose father suffered a heart attack at the age of 35 and died eight years later. Rehabilitation of a tennis injury motivated Fixx to start running to the point that he completed several marathons and even went on to write a bestselling book on running. Unfortunately, Fixx ignored the chest pains that blighted him as he ran over long distances, hoping they would eventually go away if he kept training. His passion for running came to a sad end along a road in Vermont in 1984 when Jim died of a massive heart attack in the middle of a run. An autopsy later found a complete blockage in one of his main coronary arteries, an 80% blockage in another, and signs of previous heart attacks. This event finally convinced the scientific world and the running community that running could in fact be dangerous, particularly in the case of extreme distances like the marathon.

There are of course many individual factors that contribute to the risk of running, including the underlying health of the runner, the conditions on the day, the race route, and the first aid capabilities at hand should an unfortunate emergency take place. Reviewing the data from races across the globe over the last few decades, the estimated risk of death from running is roughly 1 per 150,000 runners for the full marathon and 40% lower in those running the half marathon. These sudden events typically occur towards the end of the race or on completion, so it is thought that perhaps the surge in adrenaline, which pushes runners faster and harder nearer the finish line, could be an underlying factor. Broadly speaking, undiagnosed congenital defects can cause cardiac death amongst younger runners and contribute to coronary heart disease amongst the older community.

Jim Peters is undoubtedly one of the most famous long distance runners of all times. In the 1950s, he broke the men's record four times and was the first to complete the marathon in under 2 hours 20 minutes, a feat comparable to the four-minute mile. And perhaps most memorable of all is the 1954 Empire Games (later to be called the Commonwealth Games) held in Vancouver. Roger Bannister had just achieved the first ever four-minute mile that year and was seated in the arena awaiting the medal ceremony with his arch rival John Landy (the only other man to have broken the same barrier at that time) as the men's marathon neared completion. The stalwart and race favourite Peters entered the stadium for the finish a whole 17 minutes ahead of his nearest competitor and the race was surely to be his. But fate had a different plan for him that day. In the height of the midday sun at the hottest time of the year, the men's marathon distance had been miscalculated and was much longer than the prescribed length.

In addition to this deadly combination, the race officials near the finish line were absent from their posts as they were watching the Bannister-Landy duel, so nobody was present to inform Peters of his huge lead and the need for him to slow down. Peters therefore pushed himself harder and harder towards the finish line. As he entered the stadium to a raucous applause, he began to wobble. There were only 380 yards to go. When he first fell over, he didn't understand what was happening. His thought was that he didn't want to disgrace his wife and family and so he drove himself on. *"I could see that tape in front of my eyes, but as I got up and ran, it didn't seem to get any nearer."*

Over the next eleven minutes, Peters got up and fell several times, covering a distance of only 200 metres. He finally collapsed and lost consciousness just a few hundred yards short of the finish line. Agonising video footage of the race shows him running as though he had suffered a loss of motor control on his right hand side. He was rushed to hospital, put in an oxygen tent and given saline intravenously, and there he stayed for several days. Roger Bannister, who had just qualified as a doctor, remained in Vancouver to look after him. It is thought that his motor incoordination was the result of an encephalopathy (inflammation of the brain) brought on by his high core temperature, severe dehydration, deranged blood chemistry and lack of glucose.

So let us begin our run along the famous Mumbai Marathon and take a closer look at our incredible human physiology which changes on a second by second basis along this long journey.

## The Start Line

It's just past 5:30 am, the race is moments away from beginning and thousands of runners have lined up to participate on this cool winter's morning. Held on the third Sunday of January each year, the Mumbai Marathon is the largest marathon in Asia and the largest mass participation sporting event on the continent (as well as the greatest in terms of prize money!). Having trained rigorously for the past six months, our runner, dressed in bright, loose and minimal clothing, woke up more than two hours ago and had a light carbohydrate snack and some bananas to load some last minute energy into his bloodstream. He drank some water but was wary of filling his bladder too much on this big day. As a last-ditch attempt to lighten himself before the start, he also spent considerable time in the bathroom emptying his bowels as the last thing he wants is to make a toilet stop along the route. The night was filled with a mix of excitement, nerves and anticipation as he tried to get at least five to six hours of sleep before his first ever race. With stretching and warm up done, our hero is moments away from beginning as the ten-second countdown began. At eight seconds, his palms are clammy as the adrenaline has started to pour into his system, six and his heart begins to race, three and his mind begins to single in on the one task he now needs to undertake over and over again for the next four hours or so, one and it's all about running. The siren blows and the run begins!

In Chapter 1, I discussed the importance of oxygen and how our body captures these diatomic molecules from the air and transports them via the bloodstream to our muscles and cells. In many ways this knowledge forms a good foundation for some of the in-depth changes we will be observing in this chapter, as once again the core focus lies in understanding the engineering feats carried out by our physiological systems as they attempt to pump more blood (and with it oxygen and fuel) to our muscles to keep us going.

The first main system that we will be looking at is the cardiorespiratory system, a complex network that involves the heart, lungs and the millions of blood vessels penetrating our muscles. In the seconds before we start running, our intelligent bodies 'know' that a period of intense activity is about to begin. In those moments, a message gets sent to the vagus nerve (the tenth cranial nerve innervating the heart, lungs and gastrointestinal tract) to stop its normal inhibitory action on the heart rate. The heart, as we all know, is a muscular pump whose main action is to propel blood around the body. To do so, its own muscle is made up of a type of cell called the cardiac myocyte. The elegant feature of these cells is that unlike other kinds of muscle cells (smooth and skeletal), myocytes have their own ability to contract. That is, they beat on their own accord! The mechanism for this is very similar to the generation of nerve action potentials we learnt about in Chapter 2. Dissimilar to other muscle cells that need to be 'wired in' to a nerve and an originator box to contract, these myocytes will happily beat away even if they are isolated and placed in a dish with the right nutrients. A beautiful physiological adaptation once again by nature! Another key feature of these heart cells is that they are able to link up with one another and work in harmony to transmit electrical beats or contract in a smooth and coordinated manner. They do this by adopting the rate of the fastest beating cell amongst them. Therefore, if we were to put ten of these myocytes in a row, rather than all ten of them beating at their own individual rates, they will synchronise based on the rhythm set by the fastest myocyte, thereby passing the contractions from one end to the other. I think this is very cool, but maybe that's just me being geeky!

With this in mind, the heart which is made of millions of these myocytes has a group of specialised cells located in its right atrium (its upper chambers) called the sinoatrial node. This is the heart's natural pacemaker and as its cells beat marginally faster than the other cells of the heart, it determines how fast the heart should contract, which is roughly 100 beats per minute (bpm). You may ask why, if that is the case, healthy adults have resting heart rates of about 60–70 bpm. Indeed that's a reasonable inquiry to make. You see, in addition to its intrinsic value, the heart rate is also a product of the interplay between the sympathetic nervous system (which acts to speed it up) and the parasympathetic nervous system (which acts to slow it down). Under conditions of normality and rest, it is the parasympathetic system — through the action of the vagus nerve — that is the predominant system of the two. This vagal inhibition is the reason our heart rates are lower at rest and the fitter you are generally, the stronger the effect of this vagus outflow and hence the lower the resting pulse rate.

In the moments before exercise begins, the vagal 'tone' is removed and the heart rate jumps to its intrinsic rate of near 100 bpm. This immediate increase in heart rate raises the cardiac output, a measure of the volume of blood (in litres) that is pumped around the body per minute. The cardiac output is the product of the heart rate and the volume of blood in every heartbeat, which is called the stroke volume. At rest, this value rises from around 5 litres/min to near 25 litres/min during exercise.

As our runner began running, his cardiac output immediately jumped due to the rise in his heart rate. The mechanism for this rise is multifactorial. Interestingly, the body knew that it was going to be put under strain and therefore prepared itself by raising the heart rate. There is additionally a 'feed-forward' mechanism that is thought to exist which manifests itself through the action of mechanoreceptors. These are receptors in the joints and muscles and when they sense large movements like those during running, they send nerve impulses to the central command centre for cardiovascular control within the brain, which responds with support by increasing the heart rate.

Our maximal heart rate can be roughly calculated by subtracting one's age in years from 220. Therefore, a forty year-old man can expect his maximal rate to be approximately 180 bpm. Heart rate increases directly as a function of exercise intensity, until one reaches the point of exhaustion. As that point is approached, your heart rate begins to level off. Hence, the maximum rate is the highest heart rate value one can achieve in an all-out effort until the point of exhaustion. This is a highly reliable value that remains constant from day to day and changes only slightly from year to year. Within a few minutes of the race, our runner has more or less reached a regular cadence for his running stride and his heart rate has now reached its steady state for that level of running intensity. Should he decide to sprint a section or go up a steep slope, then the increase in requirement of blood flow will raise his rate further (provided he is still below his maximal rate).

The runner's heart rate was not the only thing that climbed in the starting seconds of the race. The same receptors that sensed movement in the joints and sent a message to the brain also resulted in a similar message being relayed to the respiratory centre, causing the runner's lungs to work harder as he increased his rate and depth of breathing. This breathing centre also reduced the resistance in the blood vessel walls of the tiny capillaries which engorge the alveoli (refer to Chapter 1) and allowed for a more efficient gas exchange in the lung substance. This cardiorespiratory 'coupling' results in an increased ventilation of close to 15 times that of our normal rate at rest.

## Mile 3 / Kilometre 5

Having left the imperial gothic structure of the world heritage Victoria Terminus train station behind him and now running along the route leading to the coastline, our runner has just turned onto Marine Drive, which is also known as the 'Queen's necklace'. A three-mile stretch of sea-hugging road, this is one of the city's iconic features and a wonderful breeze blows over the Arabian Sea, cooling the participants as they press forward. Well and truly in his stride now, our runner has been going for around 20 minutes and the body has begun its adaptive processes to tackle the workload placed upon it.

We saw the immediate changes in the runner's cardiorespiratory system as he first began to run. While this first phase was dominated by the parasympathetic system, the next phase — the prolonged stabilisation or maintenance phase — is dominated by the sympathetic system. This system is primarily controlled by the secretion of various hormones and other chemical messengers into the bloodstream, after which they exert their effects on different parts of the cardiovascular system. We first encountered its two main hormones, noradrenaline and adrenaline, in Chapter 1; here, we will build on that foundation to understand their actions in greater detail.

These chemical messengers act via specialised receptors called 'adrenoreceptors' to produce their different effects on different organs. These receptors are broadly divided into two main types, the alphas and the betas. The important thing to know about this system is that it is highly specific. Ingeniously once again, the body has created a way in which a limited number of variables can have profoundly different yet specific outcomes, independent of each other, depending on which outcome is required. Broadly speaking, the noradrenaline release targets the alpha adrenoreceptors in different vascular beds to alter the blood flowing through. This is not a one size fits all approach and the human body is able to control the amount of blood flow to each of its organs as required.

First, the degree of sympathetic outflow varies for different types of organs. Next, the number of receptors in the various organs are different, altering the dose response curve. Third, the affinity of the receptors change in different parts of the body even for the same messenger, thereby tweaking the type of response that is possible. Finally, the local effects can themselves be modulated by the actions of other locally generated substances to enhance or depress the effect being generated.

Blood flow redistribution is one of the main achievements of this system in the steady phase of exercise. At rest, the 5 litres of blood being pumped around the body is roughly divided in the following manner. About half of it is sent to the gut and the kidneys, another 20% to the muscles, roughly 15% to the brain, 6% to the skin, 4% to the heart and the rest to the other parts of the body. But as the runner is now 3 to 4 miles into the race, these volumes and more importantly these ratios have changed drastically. The muscles now receive around 70% of the blood flow and the volume has jumped from around 1 litre/min to more than 12 litres/min. The gut and the kidneys have had their volumes slashed by more than half and now their ratio has fallen to around 6–7% in total. The volume to the brain remains unchanged (though naturally the percentage has dropped as an arithmetic effect), and although the proportion of blood flow to the heart remains unchanged at 4%, more importantly this volume has increased threefold to more than 750 mL per minute. Finally, the flow of blood to the skin has doubled to around 12% and the volume has jumped almost six-fold. What does this all mean? The body is doing what it does best — preserving what is important and needed urgently, like the heart, the muscles and the skin (for temperature control), and dialing back on what it doesn't require, such as food absorption and urine production.

This redistribution is achieved through the complex effects of the sympathetic hormones in the different vascular beds, resulting in constriction in organs like the kidneys and the gut and dilatation in others like the heart, lungs and muscles.

In addition to the generalised systemic effects of the hormones, the body also creates localised vasodilatory effects within muscles through the production and release of toxic metabolites which are created by the effects of cellular respiration, such as hydrogen ions, lactic acid and carbon dioxide. These noxious molecules encourage blood flow into muscles by reducing the resistance of blood vessels, thereby increasing the outflow of these substances away from the cells.

There are principally three factors that determine blood flow resistance within a vessel, specifically its diametre and length and the viscosity (thickness) of blood flowing through. Of these three, the most important physiological factor is the tiny alterations to the vessel's diametre, brought about through contraction and relaxation of the vascular smooth muscle in the blood vessel walls. First described by the 19th century French physician Poiseuille, this famous relationship (known as Poiseuille's Equation) states that, assuming constant length and viscosity, changes in the radius of a vessel has a four-fold impact on its resistance to blood flow.

As I mentioned earlier, there are two main types of adrenoreceptors and while the alpha subtype is involved in changes in the blood vessel walls, the beta group is present in the cells of the heart and lungs and bring about changes in the organs themselves. Beta 1 receptors in the heart have multiple effects which all ultimately act towards increasing the flow of blood. Situated in the walls of the cardiac muscles, these receptors respond to circulating hormones that increase the contractile force of each heartbeat, which is also known as an increased inotropic effect.

The cells pump harder and therefore push more blood around our hardworking runner's body. Second, the receptors are also present in the sinoatrial node and the pacemaker region of the heart, known as the atrioventricular node, and enhance their excitability towards electrical impulses. This increases the rate at which they can fire, thus leading to a faster heartbeat. This is termed the chronotrophic effect. And then we have the beta 2 subclass situated in the smooth muscle cells of our airways. These cause muscle cells to relax, allowing the airways to increase in diametre (thus reducing its resistance) and creating a more facilitative environment for the rapid inflow of oxygen and outflow of carbon dioxide.

I will briefly describe one last functional adaptive capability displayed by the heart, an elastic property of the cardiac myocytes — significantly modulated during exercise. We just saw that thanks to the action of the sympathetic nervous system on the heart, its ability to beat harder increases as its contractile force increases. In addition to this chemical effect on the cell, cardiac myocytes also display a physical property that allows them to beat harder when we exercise. Put simply, they are stretchy! As the force of a myocyte's contraction is directly proportional to its length, it therefore reacts to being stretched by beating harder (this effect is called Starling's Law of the heart and I am particularly fond of this as Professor Starling primarily worked at University College London where I completed my medical and physiology degrees). So how does this help our runner? Well, as the cardiac output increases due to the many effects described above, the amount of blood flowing back to the heart also increases. This increased 'preload' physically stretches the heart muscle. In turn, the heart responds proportionately by beating harder to eject the blood out of the system. This increase in stroke volume reinforces all the various effects we have seen, working harmoniously to allow our dear runner to continue on his merry way and supplying his muscles with the oxygen and fuel it so desperately needs.

## Mile 8 / Kilometre 13

The race is now entering a very interesting phase with a significant distance already covered. Individual differences in fitness levels start to show as the stronger runners begin to lead the pack while the lesser abled slowly fall to the rear. The route saw two gentle undulations around the Peddar Road area, after which the competitors raced past the historic Haji Ali mosque that lays out at sea, connected only by a very small path that is washed over during high tide. Our runner is coping well and has been cleverly drinking small sips of water routinely throughout the race so far, replacing his water loss and aiding the body's maintenance of fluid balance, which is so vital for temperature and blood pressure control. He is just about to step on to the iconic Bandra-Worli Sea Link, a three-mile stretch of toll road built over the sea and parallel to the coast line. It is a great piece of architectural design and one of the shining stories of India's development. The road connects the Southern residential locality of Worli with the Northern district of Bandra and is simply a joy to drive on and an even bigger joy to run on (only permitted on marathon day!).

It would be useful at this point to take a step back and reflect on the concept of running. Running is more than simply walking fast. In fact, the two actions are hardly the same. When we walk, one foot is on the ground at all times. In contrast, during our running stance, we achieve a moment of aerial grace lasting around 0.12 seconds in which we are essentially flying. It is assumed that ancestral humans developed the ability to run for long distances about 2.6 million years ago, perhaps in order to hunt animals.

And although modern conditions no longer require us to run long distances in order to acquire food, competitive running as we do now initially grew out of religious festivals in various parts of the world. Records of competitive racing date back to the Tailteann Games in Ireland in 1829 B.C. while the first recorded Olympic Games took place in 776 B.C.!

Without delving too much into the mechanical nature of running and the forces acting on our body that propel us horizontally forward at speed, it would be good to take a closer look at how our muscles work. By understanding its physiology and the biochemical processes that take place in order for us to achieve running movement, we can better appreciate why we tire and how we can train more effectively to become better runners (something our subject no doubt did in order for him to reach a physiological state that is capable of attempting and completing a marathon).

The mechanical act of running exclusively involves our skeletal muscles. Under voluntary control by the brain, they gain their scientific name 'striated' due to the underlying physiological mechanisms that cause them to contract. Muscles can contract in many different ways, and interestingly not all of them involve a shortening of length. In fact, there are cases where a contracting muscle actually stays the same length or even lengthens. Already on a few occasions in this book, we have seen the importance of the action potential and the role it plays in propagating nerve impulses. So how does this electrochemical message arriving via a nerve to a muscle get converted into a force of movement? Well, an elegant mechanical explanation put forward by yet another UCL Professor of Physiology, Dr. Andrew Huxley, is the sliding filament theory.

The basic contractile unit of a muscle cell is known as the sarcomere. These are long and thin protein structures of perhaps 2–3 microns (micrometre) in length. If we were to wrap a few hundred of them together like a bundle of rope and then line up that bundle end-to-end with a few thousand other sarcomere bundles, you've just made yourself a single muscle cell or fibre. Every muscle consists of many muscle fibres, and therefore of many millions of sarcomeres. Sarcomeres are composed of two main proteins, called actin and myosin, which are neatly arranged in arrays giving muscle its characteristic striated appearance. Bands of actin, the thinner of the two proteins, form the outer scaffold of the unit, whereas myosin, the thicker filament, forms bands that interdigitate with actin. It is the conformational shape change of this molecule that creates the shortening of the sarcomere. A way to imagine this movement is to lay out your hands in front of you with both palms faced towards your chest. Now bring them into opposition with one another such that your right forefinger lays in the space between your left forefinger and middle finger, your right middle finger between your left middle and ring fingers, and your right ring finger between your left ring and little fingers. As you bring your hands together such that the tips of your fingers approach the palm line, this represents the movement of the actin and myosin against one another and the contracting muscle!

So let's home in on how this movement occurs in muscle. As the action potential of the nerve that supplies the muscle reaches its motor end plate (the large and complex terminal formation by which the axon of a motor neuron establishes synaptic contact with a striated muscle fibre), it causes the release of tiny calcium ions into the network of tubules around the muscle fibre cells. The calcium then binds to a third type of protein called tropomyosin, which is present on the actin-containing thin filaments of the myofibrils. Under normal circumstances, the tropomyosin physically obstructs the binding sites for myosin; however, once the calcium enters the cell, it frees up this site and now the two main proteins can interact and bind with one another. As these sites become available, myosin utilises a molecule of energy (ATP), binds to the actin and undergoes a 'power stroke', thus pushing the actin filaments further along its length (similar to your fingers moving towards each other in the analogy above). When I think of the power stroke, I imagine millions of tiny oarsmen. The beat of the oars is the movement of one protein against the other and this results in the contraction. After this movement, a new molecule of ATP comes and binds to the myosin head which disengages it from its binding site and returns it to its natural state. This breakdown triggers the power stroke once more and the molecules are moved along again, and thus the cycle continues. The beauty of this relationship is a little like that of quantum theory and general relativity. Physicists have been trying to marry these two main theories, one of the gigantic and the other of the minuscule, together for decades. For physiologists and scientists, the sliding filament theory does exactly that — it uses the microscopic world of proteins and molecules to explain the large movements in our sometimes metre-long muscles!

Have you ever wondered how the same action with different intended outcomes (such as throwing a ball either a short, medium or long distance) and which utilises the same muscle groups can be achieved without conscious control? This amazing capability is achieved by the body through a process called muscle activation or recruitment. We already saw that a motor unit consists of one motor neuron and all the muscle fibres it stimulates. Moreover, our muscles consist of a number of these motor units, with its fibres dispersed and intermingling amongst fibres of other units. In some cases, the muscle fibres belonging to one motor unit can in fact be spread throughout the entire muscle. Elwood Henneman, an American neurophysiologist, developed a theory known as the

Size Principle of Muscle Contraction. He stated that muscle fibres are recruited sequentially based on the need for them. *The lower the demand, the fewer fibres required, whereas the greater the demand, the more fibres required.* When the message reaches our arm to throw the ball and the corresponding sets of motor neurons are activated, all the muscle fibres innervated by that motor neuron are stimulated and then contract. The activation of one motor neuron will result in a weak but distributed muscle contraction, resulting in the ball being thrown a short distance. The activation of more motor neurons will result in more muscle fibres being activated, and therefore a stronger muscle contraction and a farther throw. Motor units are generally recruited from smallest to largest, and thus slower to faster twitches, as the contraction increases. This concept of motor unit recruitment is thus a simple measure of how many motor neurons are activated for a particular activity by a particular muscle, and is therefore also a measure of how many fibres of that muscle are needed to execute that action. The greater the recruitment, the stronger the muscle contraction will be.

Most of us would already be familiar with the fact that there are two types of muscle fibres which are classified roughly by their appearance. The first, called Type 1 fibres or 'red muscle', is also known as slow twitch fibres. These muscles are called red muscle because of the abundance of capillaries which engorge the muscle with ample blood supply and plenty of oxygen. They also house millions of energy-producing mitochondrial units that burn carbohydrate sugars and fats and hence can sustain prolonged activity — perfect for running marathons! The second variant, called Type 2 fibres or 'white muscle', can also be called the fast twitch fibres. These are more pale in comparison as they do not have as rich a blood supply network and lack the concentrated presence of mitochondria. However, they are excellent at producing short bursts of powerful activity and are thus the fibre of choice in activities like sprinting or weightlifting. The physical lack of blood and oxygen also results in these fibre types opting for an anaerobic biochemical pathway in energy production (something we will return to later on in this chapter). It is also important to stress that inference to the speed of the muscle does not relate to the speed of contraction; rather, it describes the speed at which the muscle tires. *"Give me a muscle biopsy and I'll tell you whether you should be a sprinter or a marathon runner"* is a well-known citation from sport physiologists. The organisation of these types of fibres in each of us is predominantly determined genetically — athletes with a larger proportion of Type I fibres do not make for fast runners, but are able to endure activity levels longer than those with a dominance of white fibres. The latter athletes are quicker, but their fuel stores are drained faster. That being said, all is not lost if you want to be the next Usain Bolt and a muscle biopsy finds that you have more of the Type 1, red, and slow twitch variety than the other. Studies have now shown that training can influence the variability and distribution of these muscle types and can in fact go a long way towards helping you achieve your potential.

Any reader wading through the academic literature or reading health magazines would be inundated with the sheer number of articles and writeups discussing the conversion of slow to fast twitch and vice versa. In my opinion, the real answer is likely to be more complicated than any of them make it out to be. One possible mechanism with which this effect is achieved is through the presence of a third type of muscle fibre called Type 2A or the intermediate fibre. When viewed under the microscope, these fibres are a mix between the reds and the whites and have a scattering of qualities from each type. This group of fibres are the most plastic and can transform into a redder or a whiter state. Thus, they can help athletes achieve their ideal composition. Some studies also highlight that while the overall fibre type cannot change completely, they can subtly alter themselves to resemble one type or the other more and therefore also contribute to increased performance in the intended activity domain. Hence, frequent long distance running does help to mould the intermediate 2A fibres towards the redder side of fibre anatomy and additionally increase the size, proficiency and efficiency of existing Type 1 fibres. Overall, the body's ability to run long distances is improved.

## Mile 15 / Kilometre 24

Well over halfway through the run, our star athlete has already been hard at it for over two hours. The race has entered the return leg of its loop around southern Mumbai and the runners are making their way through the residential area of Worli. Approaching 7:30 am, the sun has just risen over the horizon, splashing an orange hue against the bright blue backdrop of the sky. The temperature is a comfortable 16 degrees Celsius and there is an eastwards sea breeze cooling the runners during this difficult phase. Getting to this point in the run is no mean feat. The average fit and healthy individual would have given up by this stage had they been made to run this distance outside the confines of a dedicated training regime. As our runner continues his effort, he begins to approach his body's natural physiological limit for cardiovascular endurance, a term given by scientists to refer to an individual's VO2 max (a term we briefly saw in Chapter 1 when we considered the climber's maximal performance capability near the summit of Mt. Everest).

Otherwise known as maximal or peak oxygen uptake, VO2 max is the maximum rate of oxygen consumption as measured during incremental exercise most typically on a motorised treadmill. Reflecting the aerobic physical fitness of the individual, it is an important determinant of endurance capacity during prolonged, sub-maximal exercise. The average untrained healthy male will have a VO2 max of approximately 35–40 mL/(kg·min), while the average untrained healthy female will score approximately 27–30 mL/(kg·min). These scores can improve with training and decrease with age, although the degree of change is highly variable. A period of intense training can double the VO2 max for some individuals but will never improve it for others. In sports such as long-distance running where intense oxygen delivery and utilisation is necessary for success, athletes can record scores of up to 80–90 mL/(kg·min). We have already learnt through the previous chapters about the factors that influence the volume of oxygen consumption, which for the sake of simplicity are classified as either supply or demand. The supply side is the transport of oxygen from the lungs to the mitochondria (including lung diffusion at the alveoli, stroke volume and cardiac output, circulating blood volume, and the capillary density of the skeletal muscle). This is sometimes referred to as presentation theory. The demand side is reflected in the rate at which the mitochondria can 'reduce' oxygen (a physical reaction in which atoms gain an electron) in a process called oxidative phosphorylation, also referred to as utilisation theory. Of these two theories, the supply factor is often considered to be the limiting one. However, it has also been argued that while trained subjects are probably supply limited, untrained subjects can indeed have a demand limitation in which their cells' powerhouse units are unable to metabolise fuel and oxygen fast enough to provide efficient energy production.

So how is VO2 max measured and more importantly, what is its relevance to the body's underlying physiological systems? Accurate measurement of one's VO2 max requires an all-out effort performed under a strict protocol usually on a treadmill or bicycle in a sports performance centre. These protocols involve specific increments in the speed and intensity of the exercise and the measurement of the amount and concentration of oxygen in inhaled and exhaled air. This allows us to determine how much oxygen the athlete is using during his or her activity. What we see when this is measured, is that an individual's oxygen consumption rises linearly, as the intensity of the workout increases. But only up to a point; where after the oxygen consumption plateaus off despite increasing the exercise intensity. This plateau phase marks the VO2 max. For those of you who have had the unpleasant experience of having your own VO2 max measured, you will know just how painful it is to reach the point at which one shifts from aerobic metabolism to the anaerobic form. From this point on, it's not long before your muscle fatigue forces you to stop exercising. This test usually takes between 10 to 15 minutes and ideally requires a person to be completely rested beforehand and motivated to endure the pain long enough to find the true VO2 max! I must thank my old friend and dear colleague, Dr. Lygeri Dimitriou, Senior Lecturer of Sport Sciences at Middlesex University, for all the times she subjected (read tortured) me on her exercise bikes in the Human Performance Lab; first in preparation for the Everest expedition and then for our expedition to the Arctic Circle. I can't even count the number of times I have had to throw up in the washrooms post the VO2 max testing.

Under normal circumstances, fat and carbohydrate stores are the primary fuels that our bodies utilise during exercise. The degree to which each of these fuels acts as the primary or secondary source of energy and the efficiency of energy utilisation depends on the prior nutritional state of the individual as well as the intensity and duration of the exercise. At lower levels of prolonged exercise, most of our energy requirements come from fat. At higher intensities, carbohydrate begins to play a greater role but is limited in its duration of action. Proteins, on the other hand, play only a very small role and mainly at very high levels of energy utilisation. Let us now examine the different fuel storage systems in the body and the way they are cleverly balanced and managed to achieve the optimal energy requirement for a particular activity. Energy as we all know is extracted from the foods we eat and converted to chemical energy stored as ATP. This high-energy bond can be used in a number of biochemical reactions as a fuel with the conversion of ATP to adenosine diphosphate (ADP). As ADP begins to accumulate in our muscles, an enzyme is activated to break down a substance called phosphocreatine (PCr) which, when combined with ADP, restores our previous ATP levels. This mechanism is called the phosphagen system. The stores of PCr however are extremely limited and this system can only support muscles for about 10 seconds. Because ATP is provided from other sources as well, PCr therefore ends up being a major energy source in the first few seconds of strenuous exercise and is the main source of fuel consumption in intense exercises such as sprinting, jumping, lifting and throwing — think Usain Bolt breaking the world 100 m sprint record on finals night at London in 2012!

As we progress to more moderate forms of exertion, the body switches to carbohydrate stores to undergo aerobic and anaerobic metabolism. Under conditions of oxygen scarcity, carbohydrates go through the anaerobic pathway in which glucose is converted to lactate and 4 molecules of ATP. If there is plenty of oxygen available, the pyruvate from glucose is converted to carbon dioxide and water in the mitochondria and releases 38 molecules of ATP instead (but after accounting for inefficiencies of the system due to leakages and the energy required to undergo this change, the true output is lower at around 28–30 molecules of ATP).

Although aerobic metabolism (the oxygen-rich product of ATP) supplies energy more slowly than anaerobic metabolism, it can be sustained for long periods of time and is perfect for an activity such as marathon running. However, the major advantage of the less efficient anaerobic pathway is that it produces ATP more rapidly by utilising local stores of carbohydrates in the form of muscle glycogen. Other than PCr, this pathway is the fastest way to resupply ATP to muscles. Hence, anaerobic glycolysis supplies most of our energy needs for short-term intense exercise which typically ranges anywhere from 30 seconds to two minutes — think Michael Phelps breaking the swimming record for the 400 m freestyle race at the Sydney Olympics!

The disadvantage of this form of metabolism is that it cannot be sustained for very long periods due to the production and accumulation of lactic acid in muscle. This lactate decreases the acidity of the surrounding tissues and deactivates key enzymes involved in the glycolysis pathway, leading to what we colloquially describe as having a 'stitch' which is actually muscle fatigue. This lactic acid then needs to be circulated via the bloodstream to the liver where it is converted to glycogen and stored again for reuse at a later point. The stored glycogen in our muscles is the preferred carbohydrate fuel for sports lasting less than two hours for both aerobic and anaerobic metabolism. As we have learnt, the depletion of muscle glycogen causes fatigue and is associated with a buildup of lactic acid. This lactate production increases continuously, but physiologists have defined a point at which our breathing changes as a direct result of acid-base imbalance in our muscles and blood and have termed it the anaerobic threshold.

## Mile 20 / Kilometre 32

He stumbles. His vision begins to narrow. He feels delirious and wobbly as though his legs are turning into jelly. All of a sudden, he is faced with his first doubt of being able to complete this race which he trained so long and hard for. It doesn't help that he has the return leg of the hill on Peddar Road to complete and his legs are increasingly heavy and immovable. He slows and almost stops but wills himself to keep going. Our runner is experiencing what we colloquially call 'bonking', also otherwise known as hitting the wall!

The scientific explanation for this event is the condition caused by the depletion of glycogen stores in the liver and muscles during intense prolonged exercise, which manifests itself as sudden loss of energy and fatigue. We have already learnt that glycogen is our body's main source of energy during exercise. Most of us have around 380 grams of it stored in our muscles and livers, which roughly equates to about 1500 kcal of energy. The average runner burns between 600–800 kcal per hour during the run, so we would expect our internal source of energy (glycogen) to run out anywhere between two to three hours, which is exactly what is happening to our athlete. What is also of interest is that regular long distance exercises can actually increase the total amount of stored fuel in our bodies so that we are progressively able to achieve longer and longer distances (up to a point!).

Such fatigue can become seriously debilitating and the symptoms include general weakness, severe fatigue, and the various manifestations of hypoglycemia which, when mild, can just be dizziness, but more severe forms can include even hallucinations. The important fact is that this condition will not be relieved by brief periods of rest and must include carbohydrate replacements. For this very reason many runners consume small doses of sugary drinks, bananas and sweet jellies or natural substitutes — all with the aim of delaying the point at which the wall is reached. To make matters worse, scientists also claim that the brain's production of dopamine, the happy hormone responsible for generating feelings of excitement, reward, motivation, and pleasure, begins to drop. In turn, this may produce the negative mental voices in our heads telling us that we can't do it. As our runner meanders and wobbles on, he forces himself to consume more sugars handed out to him by the supportive crowd along the route. A small banana, a few sweets, a sugary drink and some water later, his will begins to return and he is once again able to focus his mind on the finish line. This helps him overcome the pain signals being released from each and every corner of his body. He has worked so hard to prepare for this run and he is not going to give up. Adrenaline surges, the glycolytic pathways kick back into action and he powers on along the road.

His muscles are at the point of fatigue. The development of muscle fatigue is typically defined as a reduction in the maximal force of our muscles. However, this also means that contractions, although suboptimal, can still be sustained despite the onset of fatigue. There is even evidence that activities involving muscles other than the principal ones can continue working. The metabolic buildup of noxious substances within the muscles (like chloride, potassium and lactate) and the diminishing of the substrate required to maintain contractions (i.e., glycogen) are the two main factors behind this tiring. The generation of inadequate commands from his motor cortex in the brain also contributes to his increased fatigue. An interesting theory which has been in circulation for the past fifteen years is the Central Governor Model of fatigue. It puts the brain at the centre of all our activities and suggests that exercise is regulated based on a neurally calculated 'safe exertion level', such that our level of physical activity is controlled so that its intensity cannot threaten the body's ability to stay alive. The brain limits our ability to exercise by shutting off the neuronal signals sent to our muscles to make them contract when it believes that our body as a whole may be at risk. Put forward by Professor Noakes from Cape Town University, he postulated that *"the power output by muscles during exercise is continuously adjusted in regard to calculations made by the brain in regard to a safe level of exertion. These neural calculations factor in earlier experience with strenuous exercise, the planning duration of the exercise, and the present metabolic state of the body. These brain models ensure that body homeostasis is protected, and an emergency reserve margin is maintained. This neural control adjusts the number of activated skeletal muscle motor units, a control which is subjectively experienced as fatigue. This process, though occurring in the brain, is outside personal control"*. In his view, fatigue is in many ways like an emotion which has no functional characteristics other than the tendency to make us want to stop. The generation of this overwhelming desire to slow down and cease effort is our body's way of protecting us from the harm caused by remaining in a state of heightened activity. For those of you who run or indulge in long duration intense activities, I am sure you can relate to this phenomena whereby even though all you want to do is to keep going and achieve your goal, your body or rather your mind is just unable to overcome the physical desire to stop and rest.

## Mile 26 / Kilometre 42

He is just a few hundred yards short of the finish line. Five hours of running has taken its toll on the runner. His feet, legs, back and head all pound with immense pain. He has had to fight all his mental demons in order to keep moving his legs one in front of the other, over and over again. Every time his foot hits the ground, a stress three to four times his body weight is absorbed by his ankles, knees, hips, and lower back. And with each stride, some muscles contract to propel the body forward while others contract to control the degree of movement by being lengthened. These eccentric lengthening contractions are notorious for damaging the muscle's infrastructure and will result in a week or more of pain once he finishes. But for now, as he sees the façade of the historic and world-famous Victoria Terminus train station come into view, he knows the end point is near. Built in 1887 to commemorate the golden jubilee of Queen Victoria and relic of the British Raj, the impressive gothic structure is among the most beautiful in India. The finish line with its towering digital clock lay metres in front of him and he lifts his arms to the heavens as he completes the last few strides across the line. Tears well up in his eyes as he is overpowered by emotions, and as if in slow motion, he collapses to the ground. It's as though his legs just said enough is enough and refused to budge another inch. Fortunately, a warm reception of friends and fellow runners help him to his feet and support him to a place to rest and recover. What a journey it has been!

The long road to recovery for our runner is just about to begin. His muscles and bones will now begin the physiological work of repairing themselves from the heavy impact of this run. Tears in his musculature and tendons and microfractures in his weight-bearing bones will reroute his body's resources to try and restore them. Biochemically, his metabolism will remain in a heightened state of activity for the next few days. His immune system will also be weakened, thus making him prone to viral illnesses, and his cardio-vascular system will need a period of rest to adjust itself back from this sustained activity. All this being said, it could indeed very well be true that there is no other sport in the world that is so popular and yet has such potentially harmful effects as marathon running. Decades (if not more) of studies on runners indicate that the phys-iological stresses of running these 26-odd miles far out-weigh the physiological benefits to the body. At best, the successful marathon runner will have a few thousand calories less to carry around with him and once the recovery process is over, a stronger heart, bones and muscles will result. But from my own experience of marathon running, I feel that the real benefits are actually psychological and emotional in nature. Despite the fact that running a marathon is hard on the body, from a scientist's standpoint, every runner who crosses that finish line has personally attested to the miracle that is the human body!

I will never forget my first full marathon finish. As I approached the penultimate kilometre, to see my wife, my family and friends (with all their little children) screaming my name and holding up signs of support, my physical spirit lifted. They ran alongside me for the last kilometre, with my son Aeden in front of me. I went off ahead for the last 100 metres, wanting to cross the finish line alone. With every ounce of strength I could muster, I raised my arms in the air as I went across the line, flooded with emotion. Not because of the sixteen years of dreaming or the five months of sacrifice I had made to get here. But to know that this day marks the start of something new. That forever more, I will be a Marathon finisher. That forever more I will live unconstrained by my physical limits. That forever more, borrowing the words of a running legend, I will live knowing that I AM POSSIBLE.

# 4 The Red Planet

"It suddenly struck me that that tiny pea, pretty and blue, was the Earth. I put up my thumb and shut one eye, and my thumb blotted out the planet Earth. I didn't feel like a giant. I felt very, very small."

— **Commander Neil Armstrong**

'Boom!' I heard Atlantis fire her rockets and I was immediately enveloped in a powerful thunderous wave that shook me to my core. It was like an incredibly fast drum roll, one which gets faster and louder, like nothing I had ever experienced before. An astronaut once described a shuttle launch as 'it seems the air just isn't big enough for the sound'. Even though the space shuttle was just under two miles away from me, the force with which is pushed back against the Earth to lift it up off the pad physically shook the very ground beneath my feet; just imagine what her crew must have been feeling at that point in time. Wave after wave of supersonic sound generated by her engines spread through the sky. Every organ within me vibrated to the sound of her engines. She started slowly at first but then began to tear away faster and faster into the blue sky. Momentarily Atlantis disappeared behind a plume of fluffy white cumulus clouds but her bright orange tail of fire lit up the sky like a torch. We all looked at each other in sheer amazement as she continued on upwards and eastwards.

— Personal diary excerpt, Mission STS-122,
Kennedy Space Centre (N.A.S.A), 2008

The date was 20th July 1969 and it was dinner time on the East Coast of the USA. Millions of people across the country and indeed the world were glued to their TV screens as black and white images of a momentous event were being relayed through television networks. Fast approaching the surface of the Moon, a tiny spacecraft serving as the landing module of the Apollo 11 mission dubbed the Eagle was zipping across the lunar landscape. Everything seemed on track and the late President Kennedy's speech made nine years ago was soon becoming a reality. However, four minutes before touchdown, a small light appeared on the overhead panel flashing the words 'Error 1202' and an alarm went off at the mission control station in Houston. The Eagle was only 6,000 feet above the surface and the tiny onboard computer, which had less processing power than modern day digital watches, communicated that it was overloaded with data and needed to reboot.

The 'right stuff '. What is that? If you've ever had the privilege of listening to any of the 12 brave men who have set foot and walked on a world other than our own, you'll often hear them use this phrase to describe what it takes to become an astronaut. A strength of character to overcome the most difficult of situations, the wisdom to know the right move instinctively and the ability to execute it with near perfect precision. No one had more of the right stuff than Commander Neil Armstrong. Faced with the situation of aborting the mission as well as the hopes and dreams of a nation and mankind, and with only 60 seconds of fuel left in his chamber and a landing ground completely inappropriate for touchdown, he didn't think twice. Immediately taking the ship into manual mode, using an etched grid on his port side window and barking out the vehicle's speed, pitch and altitude to his co-pilot 'Buzz' Aldrin, Armstrong had the world on the edge of their seats as he steered the Eagle towards the Sea of Tranquility (the name given to the area that the spaceship was slated to land). Rumour has it that President Nixon was prepared to address the world with the sad news of the mission's failure, but fate had a different plan for mankind that day. A minute later, a long metal rod extending from the landing legs touched the lunar plain and signaled their arrival. A blue light on the console came on — 'CONTACT LIGHT' — and the landing was over. *"Houston, Tranquility Base here… the Eagle has landed,"* Armstrong uttered these immortal words. The first two men stayed on the Moon for just under 22 hours in total, spending two and half hours walking on its surface. Taking off from the Moon, the Eagle joined the Command Module piloted by Captain Michael Collins in lunar orbit and the three men arrived back home to a hero's welcome. On his return, Captain Aldrin remarked, *"This has been far more than three men on a mission to the Moon; more, still, than the efforts of a government and industry team; more, even, than the efforts of one nation. We feel that this stands as a symbol of the insatiable curiosity of all mankind to explore the unknown."*

Three years later, in the winter of 1972, the last of the Apollo missions blasted off from the Moon. With the space race with the former USSR over and the Vietnam War taking its toll on the national sentiment and, more importantly, its budget, the USA ended its manned Moon programme and we as a species have been left poorer for it. However, the last 50 years have seen us make tremendous progress as we ventured further and farther into the deep reaches of space. Voyager One, launched more than 40 years ago, become the first manmade object to reach beyond the limits of our solar system in 2012 and is now well on its way to our closest starry neighbour. We have sent probes into orbit and have landed on many of the other planets, their satellites and even comets and asteroids within our solar system. Technology has made these ships smaller and more powerful and our study of the solar system continues to expand year after year, including the search for life on a world other than our own.

Arguably, creating a permanent human presence in low orbit around our planet is mankind's biggest achievement in the last two decades. Visible with the naked eye in the night sky, the International Space Station (ISS) is 350 feet long and 250 feet wide and circumnavigates the Earth 15 times a day. With the capacity to hold up to six crew members, the ISS is our first permanent outpost beyond our world and in many ways will be our stepping stone to many more worlds to come. Apart from a technological feat, it also acts as a symbol of international cooperation as five different international space agencies (and many more individual country-level agencies) from across the globe have come together to work on this shared vision.

Mars, the red planet — Earth's neighbour in the solar system and its closest cousin. Mankind first probed the planet in 1971 and since then dozens of missions have orbited around it or crashed or landed on its red soil. There are nine active missions on the planet at present, including two rovers (only one is still able to slowly drive across the Martian landscape and beam back amazing images of its mountains and valleys), one stationary science unit and six orbiters circling the planet, measuring its atmosphere and mapping its surface for future landings. Our study of Mars has shown it to be remarkably similar to our own home — just a few million years ahead of us in its own planetary lifespan. Vast craters and volcanoes dominate its landscape and the networks of valleys and crevasses suggest that there was abundant flowing water across its surface in the past (with some occurring transiently even today!). An estimated five million cubic kilometres of ice has also been discovered on the surface of the planet, mainly at its poles.

The eventual aim is to try and find signs of life to help us answer one of the ultimate questions of the universe, whether we are in fact alone. The exciting news is that we are finally approaching the technology and more importantly the resolve to try and send humans to its surface. The race is now on, country versus country, private industry versus governments, for a manned mission to the planet — most likely by the mid-2030s, in what would be a truly remarkable feat for our species.

It's important to comprehend the sheer scale of the task at hand. While we have already landed 12 members of our species onto a terrestrial body beyond Earth and returned them home successfully, going to the Moon represents just a fraction of the difficulty in making a round trip to Mars. Putting it into perspective, the distance from Earth to the Moon is around 380,000 km (approximately 250,000 miles). Because of its elliptical orbit, Mars is, on the other hand, 55 million km away at its closest to Earth and more than 400 million km away its farthest! While travelling to the Moon, the Apollo missions took around two to three earth days to reach orbit. Even with our advanced propulsion systems and planning capabilities today, it will take around six earth months at minimum to achieve orbit around Mars (assuming that we are capable of overcoming all the technical and engineering difficulties to launch a mission of this scale, which we are still nowhere near). Factoring in the return voyage and the necessary interplanetary alignment for the journey home on minimal fuel requirements, the current planning timelines put a round trip anywhere upwards of at least 450 Earth days. Putting this in perspective, the longest time any human has spent in space to date has been 437 Earth days by cosmonaut Polyakov onboard the Russian Mir space station, and in that time, the effects of space (which we shall learn about in this chapter) took a heavy toll on his body. You may have noticed that

I refer to time in terms of Earth days and Earth months. This is because we have become accustomed to describing time in terms of the duration taken for planet Earth to do something, such as completing a rotation around its axis or revolving around the Sun. But this does not mean that the same definition holds true for other planets or parts of the solar system. For instance, one Martian day equates to 24 hours and 39 minutes and one Martian year equates to 687 days, so space scientists strive to ensure that the unit of time is standardised based on Earth's, especially when multiple planets or moons are involved. (The real physics enthusiasts amongst you will also know that time passes at different rates in different parts of the solar system as influenced by gravity and speed, but that I shall leave for another conversation!)

Space is a dangerous place to send complicated and delicately tuned systems like our human bodies and the two main life threatening factors are the lack of gravity and exposure to radiation. Microgravity, as it is called, affects a host of human physiological systems in a very odd manner and, if left unchecked, astronauts could arrive on Mars being depressed, frail and weak, brittle-boned, and maybe even blind. It is very likely that they will be unable to maintain their blood pressure whilst standing and that their ability to land a spacecraft will be greatly diminished due to changes in their balance and coordination. This is not quite the heroic image that mankind wants to see as the first members of the human race set foot (or possibly collapse and fall) on the red planet.

A story goes that on one summer's evening in medieval England a young scientist sitting under an apple tree on the grounds of Trinity College at Cambridge was struck on his head by a fallen fruit. In that eureka moment, the young man suddenly 'discovered' gravity. While we know that this story is indeed a myth,

Sir Isaac Newton, the young man in question, first published his work on the theories of gravity in *Principia* in 1687, and this book laid the foundations for much of what we now know of this natural phenomenon. Gravity warps the fabric of space-time around itself, resulting in a force on other objects around it. The strength of this force is directly proportional to the object's size and, in particular, its mass. Small objects like cars and houses have negligible impact on the other objects around it, whereas large dense objects like the Moon and the planets have a much stronger degree of influence. This is why we don't feel the impact of this force from ordinary objects as we go about our daily lives, but it explains why the Moon goes round the Earth, why the Earth goes round the Sun and why light cannot escape a black hole. Just like how we throw a ball up in the air or an aircraft stalls in flight, objects get attracted by the gravitational effect of the Earth and are 'pulled' back towards the surface (actually towards the earth's centre). Gravity therefore exists all around us and influences us more than we realise.

Just as humans have evolved over the generations to the conditions of Earth's temperature, pressure and atmosphere, we have also evolved under the influence of its gravity. This constant force acting upon our body has crafted our physiological systems much more than we initially appreciate. Conversely, when we send humans into space where the gravitational component is removed (which we call microgravity instead of zero gravity, as zero gravity is technically impossible) or when we land humans on a terrestrial object like the Moon or Mars where their smaller masses exert a smaller gravitational force relative to Earth's, changes to the physiological systems of our bodies can be observed, all of which are symptomatic and can have debilitating long-term consequences. Studying these effects and developing ways to combat them are paramount if we are to successfully land man on far away objects involving long sojourns through space and microgravity. Later in this chapter, we will explore the main systems that undergo changes, including the heart and our many blood vessels, the systems that underlie our balance and coordination and the systems that are responsible for the creation and maintenance of our bones and muscles.

We are bathed in a sea of radiation, high speed particles and electromagnetic waves which take the form of light, television and radio waves as well as microwaves in our day-to-day lives. Beyond these also exist the ultraviolet and infrared waves occupying the two extremes of the spectrum. While the former types of waves, which are used for everyday requirements, are mostly harmless to us, the types of radiation that exist in ionising forms can be life threatening. Gamma rays, protons and neutrons are the most common ionising forms and because they move with sufficient energy to be able to remove electrons from their orbits around atoms, they are highly reactive and unstable and we need protection from them. The Sun produces a constant stream of particles which billow out into space and travel at almost 1 million miles per hour and this stream of particles, called the solar wind, varies in intensity with the amount of surface activity on the Sun. In addition to this, the background nuclear activity of the vast solar system, galaxy and universe beyond also produces various other harmful forms of radiation known as galactic cosmic radiation.

While on or at least in orbit around our home planet Earth, we are protected from these various forms of radiation either by the ozone layer in our atmosphere or by the magnetic field created around the planet by its magnetic core. The rotation of the planet's molten iron core creates an electric current that produces a protective magnetic field around the Earth, which extends several thousand kilometres out from the surface. This magnetic field shields our planet from the harmful radioactive rays emitted by the Sun and the universe, which in turn protects the fragile life on Earth. As we have seen from the many nuclear disasters that have struck humanity throughout history, radiation is devastating, be it deliberate in the cases of Hiroshima and Nagasaki during the Second World War or accidental in the recent case of the Fukushima Daiichi power plant that was destroyed by a tsunami in 2011. The cellular degradation due to damaged DNA and other key molecular structures within our cells affects their ability to divide normally, resulting in many unhealthy symptoms. These could be acute, including nausea, vomiting, burns, falling blood counts and neurological death, or chronic, leading to problems such as cataracts, severe neurological damage and cancer. Astronauts have been classified as radiation workers; thus, monitoring their radiation exposure has been a key requirement since the early days of Project Mercury.

In the medium to long term, an increase in the risk of developing cancer due to exposure to space radiation is the principal concern, and it is a risk that persists after returning to Earth. Exposure to radiation with sufficient energy, such as that which we see in space, causes ionisations of the molecules within living cells. At low doses, such as that which we receive every day from background radiation, cells can repair the damage rapidly. But at higher doses, the cells may not be able to repair themselves and can either be changed permanently or die, leading to the development of cancerous cells. To prevent this risk, mission control has developed a number of tools to mitigate both the time and the amount of exposure to radiation. This includes physical barriers to radiation such as the construction of the hull design and shielding as well as flight maneuvers to reduce the amount of time spent in high energy areas.

Vacuum is space that is devoid of matter. Whilst no environment can be a perfect vacuum due to the presence of some ions, hydrogen atoms or small particles, outer space comes closest to being a vacuum. However, the atmospheric density within the first few hundred kilometres above the Earth's surface is still sufficient to produce a significant drag on satellites, requiring most artificial satellites operating in this region (called low earth orbit) to fire their engines once every few days to maintain their orbits. This vacuum is very hazardous for life as it is devoid of the atoms we need to survive, chiefly oxygen. Humans exposed to a vacuum will lose consciousness after a few seconds and die of hypoxia within minutes. The reduction in pressure lowers the boiling temperature of blood and other bodily fluids and while blood does not boil as many movies depict, the formation of gas bubbles in our bodily fluids, known as ebullism, is a major concern. We shall meet this phenomenon again when we read about the dangers of scuba diving and the pathologies at play when we stress our bodies by reaching the depths of oceans and resurfacing in a dangerous manner.

Time and time again, Hollywood depicts the hapless astronaut exposed to space vacuum as suffering a violent and bloody death. There is often an ear-shattering symphony of screams as the increasingly bloated space traveller writhes in agony and spasms. Their exposed veins and eyeballs rapidly swell like over-inflated balloons, ultimately bursting in a gruesome blood-filled explosion. History as well as a series of accidents and experiments have however shown this movie description to be grossly inaccurate. Upon exposure to vacuum in space, a few minor incidents quickly coalesce into a life threatening cocktail. The first effect is the expansion of gases within the lungs and the digestive tract caused by the reduction of external pressure. A victim of this 'explosive decompression' can greatly increase their chances of survival by simply exhaling rapidly within the first few seconds; otherwise death will occur as the lungs rupture and spill bubbles of air into the circulatory system causing tiny air emboli. Next, in the absence of any atmospheric pressure, water molecules spontaneously convert to vapour as they boil away, starting on the exposed surfaces such as the tongue and eyes followed by the water in our blood, muscles and organs. This would cause our bodies to swell, perhaps to twice the normal size, but the skin is unlikely to break and certainly not burst. Nitrogen within our blood stream would quickly begin to form bubbles, a condition we call the 'bends' in divers which causes immense pain and neurological symptoms, and one which we will return to in a later chapter. Any direct exposure of the skin to the Sun's rays would cause immediate and severe burns and despite the intense cold, we are unlikely to freeze. A person would be estimated to have about ten seconds of useful consciousness to try and save life and limb, but any longer and the lack of air pressure will quickly result in asphyxiation as the body is completely starved of oxygen. Unconsciousness and convulsions would follow several seconds later, and a blue discolouration of the skin called cyanosis would become evident. At this point the victim would be floating in a blue, bloated and unresponsive stupor, but their brain would remain undamaged and their heart would continue to beat. These conditions can be reversed if the astronaut is supplied with fresh pressurised oxygen within a few minutes.

In order to counteract these potential dangers, mission control has over the years designed increasingly sophisticated capsules and space suits to allow humans to venture into space and once there, to emerge from womb-like spaceships and enter the orbits of other planets or walk on their surfaces like we did on the Moon. Extra vehicular activities, otherwise known more colloquially as spacewalks, are essentially a free fall from the space station or shuttle to which the astronaut is tethered to towards the planet's surface. The inherent difficulty with designing a spacecraft is that it needs to be hardy enough to withstand the forces of launching and landing, combat radiation and meteorite impact and maintain the artificial internal environment of pressure, temperature and oxygen needed by its crew; all while being as light as possible so that a rocket can lift it off the surface against the pull of gravity and position it in space with minimum energy expenditure (read: fuel). The earliest designs of the Apollo missions had lunar modules that were designed with such efficiency to be only 0.03 centimetres thin at some places, which is as thick as a sheet of paper! It's no wonder that early astronauts were paranoid about putting their feet through the walls of the spacecraft while maneuvering around at zero gravity.

My wife calls me a geek, and I suppose I am one. I've always been into science and mathematics since I was a child and although it embarrasses me to admit it, yes I love watching science fiction and yes, I am a 'Trekkie' — if you don't know what that term means, then you're probably reading the wrong book! Looking up at the night sky, it's hard not to fall in love with the immense vastness of space and the incredible realm of probabilities and possibilities that must exist out there. Sometimes I even regret being born at this time in human history when all the really hard discovery expeditions like Everest and the Poles have just been completed while the new frontiers of space exploration are still many more years to come in the future. For years I read about the amazing journeys of man as we stepped out into another world in the late 1960s and then sent out electronic messengers in the form of probes well into our current times. I dream of one day being able to walk on the Moon or looking back down on our green and blue home set against the darkness of space from the ISS. Having the chance to study the physiological impacts of space travel was a dream come true during my university years and while doing my BSc degree I was fortunate to have one of the most amazing doctors I have ever met be a lecturer and a mentor to me, Dr. Kevin Fong. In many ways it's thanks to his inspiration that I really fell in love with the subject matter and the rest is history.

It was a beautiful, cool and crisp Thursday morning on the 7th of February 2008, a day that I will never forget. The day before, I waved goodbye to seven of the bravest humans I have had the honour to be in the presence of. Suited up in their bright orange jumpsuits, they boarded a 1950s style minibus (called the Astro-van) and were escorted to launchpad 39A to ready themselves for their departure from Earth. I left my flat on Cocoa Beach earlier than usual that morning, driving along the quiet road into Kennedy Space Centre NASA and arriving for the prelaunch meeting for the medical response team. I was still only a medical student and could not believe that I was actually present at NASA along with the planners and engineers who had worked for months if not years preparing for this moment. Luckily for me, the two previous planned launches for this mission got scrubbed and I was actually going to have a chance to watch the shuttle launch live right in front of me!

It was T-minus 2 hours and I was driven to the perimetre of the launch site for space shuttle Atlantis' mission STS 122 to the ISS. This was a special mission as buried in the huge belly of Atlantis was the Columbus science laboratory, built by the European Space Agency. This module was going to be the science and research lab of the ISS and would allow mankind to continue expanding upon its existing knowledge of micro gravitational science and enhance our ability to carry out ever more complicated experiments in space. I was alongside the emergency response team and although we were the closest people allowed to the shuttle, we were still located about two miles from her due to the potential dangers of an explosion during a launch failure. The week prior, I was invited on board the towering 200 feet-high metallic launch structure. Set against the amazing blue Atlantic Ocean, Atlantis was quite a sight with its bright orange external fuel tank and twin solid rocket boosters. These rockets would eventually be filled with liquid (and solid) oxygen, hydrogen and other highly explosive fuels and catalysts, all of which would be ignited in a controlled explosion with the purpose of lifting this massive two thousand tonne machine 250 miles into Earth's orbit at 17,000 miles per hour — incredible! I walked the final gangway that our astronauts would be led down and peered through the tiny glass window on one of the hatches. Inside, engineers dressed in white were busy making final checks and preparations for next week's journey.

While in terms of distance it doesn't seem like very much, the journey from Cape Canaveral to the ISS is probably the hardest one of all from a technical precision and safety perspective. As we are all well aware, gravity acts to keep everything firmly placed on terra firma. And while we have built machines that can power us into the air, commercial aeroplanes must still come back down to earth eventually. In order to beat the planet's massive pull upon all objects, a huge amount of force is required to work against the pull of gravity. Newton's second law of motion calculates this force to be equal to the mass of the shuttle multiplied by the acceleration it needs to overcome, in this case against gravity, which acts at 9.8 metres per second. This explosive force, the effective speed at which the object needs to travel, is called the escape velocity and is roughly 17,000 miles per hour. Through the brute force of her engines, the shuttle will travel at sufficient speed to transport the crew within their module to a height for it to be considered a low earth object. At around 250 miles above the surface, many people mistakenly believe the force of gravity to be negligible and that humans along with all the other contents of a spaceship will float around freely. Instead, travelling this distance merely reduces the pull of gravity on our bodies by around 10–15%. So how is that we see these amazing images of astronauts being lighter than air swimming around in space?

We tend to think of a rocket as only travelling upwards in a straight line, but this isn't really what happens. Its perpendicular direction of travel is quickly translated into an increasingly horizontal one until the point it enters orbit and its fuel has burned out. From there on, the shuttle is in fact moving under its own momentum from the kinetic energy of the launch in a rarefied atmosphere that produces very little drag to slow it down. Atlantis will then move in a horizontal direction across the surface of the planet, orbiting Earth around 15 times a day at a speed of close to eight kilometres per second. The shuttle is in fact free falling back towards Earth, but as it is travelling so quickly in the direction of the Earth's surface, it is actually falling away at a faster rate than she can hit the surface and so the shuttle, her crew and all the objects within her end up being in orbit. In this orbital journey around the Earth's surface, our bodies are principally in a state of weightlessness and subject to the many hazards of gravitational unloading which impact the various physiological systems we shall now learn more about.

We're at 4,000 feet and air traffic control has just cleared us to begin a series of maneuvers pretty much aimed at getting me to see the contents of my breakfast again. This was my third year in the British Royal Air Force. Serving as a medic in ground branch, each time I had the chance to get some flying time in, the pilot instructors loved to try and tear into us 'land-loving' folk. I was flying a dual-seated propeller Grob Tutor aircraft, and although it looked like a recreational model plane, it was one of the most aerobatic training aircrafts available. Today's plan was simple — after a few circuits (a flight path involving take off, four right turns downwind which line you back again for finals, landing and then repeating the process again), the instructor wanted me to "feel the blood in my pants!" by running me through a series of quick ascents up to 10,000 feet with sharp turns followed by a drop back to 2,000 feet and then repeat. Air traffic control had cleared the area and we were given the green light to begin. "I have control," said the instructor, taking charge of the plane from me. He throttled up to full and pulled the yolk stick back. It felt like we were climbing vertically (we weren't but it always feels worse than it is!). He banked hard to the left at 45 degrees and then to the right again. We climbed to 6,000 feet and then repeated the same again. I felt heavy in my seat and my face felt like it was dropping, particularly my jaw. Before I knew it, we were at 10,000 feet and suddenly he looked at me, smiled and said, 'Hold on.' We nose-dived and I screamed. The blood rushed to my head and my eyes felt like they were bulging out. We carried on this exercise for the next 5–6 minutes until I pretty much begged him to stop. It was clear to me then that while I may have a passion for aviation, spaceflight and beyond, I clearly do not have the head or the stomach for it!

As I taxied the plane back to the bay, my mind began to reflect on what fighter jet pilots must be going through as they propel their body through huge G-force variations. Their descriptions of their legs becoming heavier and blood draining away from their faces became more tangible after this encounter of mine. Pilots often describe a tunnel vision effect as their field of view narrows and becomes greyer towards the periphery. In extreme cases a blackout arises and they can temporarily lose consciousness. Why this happens and the long-term effects of these changes are all down to gravity.

An important phenomenon to understand at this point is what blood pressure (BP) is, how it is controlled and what happens when it goes wrong. It's a vital measurement that is assessed so routinely in clinics and outpatient rooms that most of us take it for granted. As such, it is something most of us probably know a little about, but never fully understand. Our BP refers to the arterial pressure of our systemic circulation or the pressure exerted by circulating blood upon the walls of blood vessels and is therefore a surrogate pressure gauge for the cardiovascular system. A person's blood pressure is usually expressed in terms of the systolic pressure over diastolic pressure and is measured in millimetres of mercury (mm Hg). Our BP is situationally dependent and the normal resting blood pressure is around 120/80 mm Hg. The numerator refers to the amount of pressure in your arteries during the contraction of your heart muscle (called the systolic pressure) and the denominator refers to the arterial pressure when your heart muscle relaxes between beats (called the diastolic pressure). Hypertension, otherwise known as high BP, puts a mechanical stress on the heart and blood vessel walls and when severe and prolonged can lead to pathologies such as heart disease, strokes and hemorrhages. Low BP on the other hand is known as hypotension and can result in symptoms suggestive of poor blood perfusion, particularly in the brain which causes symptoms such as dizziness, fainting and shock. There are many physical factors that influence arterial pressure, including the blood volume which is controlled by the Renin-Angiotensin system through the actions of the kidney, the resistance (read: diametre) in blood vessel walls which we have read about in previous chapters as being controlled by secreted hormones such as adrenaline and nitric oxide, and finally the viscosity of the blood itself which can be controlled by drugs and other agents. Our body has a system of receptors known as baroreceptors which are responsible for the beat-to-beat detection of our BP and sending messages to organs like the adrenal glands, kidneys, heart and blood vessels through the action of the nervous system. These baroreceptors can control or adjust the pressure to achieve optimum levels. The most important arterial baroreceptors are located in the left and right carotid sinuses as well as the aortic arch. They send signals to the medulla in the brain stem, which adjusts the mean arterial pressure by altering both the force and speed of the heart's contractions as well as the total peripheral resistance.

The efficiency of the cardiac pump function is dependent on the gravitational field, position of the body and the functional characteristics of blood vessels. One of the most profound changes that occur immediately when exposed to zero G is the cephalad redistribution of blood caused by a lack of hydrostatic pressure. The term cephalad simply means the movement of fluid towards the head and is often witnessed in flight as astronauts appear to have puffy faces and 'chicken legs'. These appear within the first 24 hours of flight and reach a steady state within 2 to 5 days. In a constant gravitational environment, the cardiovascular system continues to deliver blood against the effects of gravity. Because humans usually maintain an upright position, 70% of our blood volume is located in the venous circulation below the level of the heart. Pooling is the term used to describe the displacement of blood away from the thorax to the peripheral veins, and this blood is not stationary but is in transit around the circulatory system. The heart normally generates a dynamic pressure with the mean pressure settling around 100 mm Hg. Two other components additionally contribute to the final blood pressure — a static pressure generated by the elastic properties of the vasculature and a hydrostatic pressure generated due the force of gravity which is equal to the density of blood ($\rho$) times the acceleration force of gravity ($g$) times the height of the vertical blood column ($h$) from the heart (i.e., $\rho \times g \times h$).

Therefore, we say that the heart pumps blood *in spite of* gravity. When we are in the supine position (i.e., lying down), there is a negligible gravitational component as the head, feet and heart are all about the same level. This mimics the conditions of microgravity. It is for this reason that Earth-based studies where subjects are asked to lay down for months on end (i.e., bed rest studies) are used as a substitute for zero-gravity studies on astronauts in outer space. In this supine position, most of our blood is concentrate around the compliant veins of the abdomen and chest. When we stand up or return to Earth, our circulatory system is suddenly exposed to gravitational stress and the hydrostatic component returns. In healthy individuals, this pooling in the legs and inadequate perfusion of the brain is monitored and controlled by the nervous system, which makes the necessary adjustments to maintain appropriate blood pressure.

Orthostatic Intolerance (OI) is one of the main adverse consequences associated with space flight under zero gravity. OI refers to a person's inability to maintain an appropriate blood pressure when made to stand from a supine position, or in the case of astronauts, to stand for 10 minutes or more. The normal response for this change is a stabilisation to the upright position in approximately sixty seconds. During this process, the normal change in heart rate would be an increase of 10 to 15 beats per minute and a 10 mm Hg increase in diastolic pressure with only a slight change in systolic pressure. These changes occur to maintain adequate blood pressure and thus adequate perfusion to the  brain. The problem with OI is that astronauts may find themselves suddenly back in a gravitational environment after having spent six months on board a spaceship to Mars. They may lose their ability to maintain BP and more importantly cerebral perfusion while standing — not an ideal scenario when landing on a new world!

The mechanisms behind OI are complex and are currently studied in great detail so that we can have a better grasp of the exact sequence of events. Broadly speaking, research has found that the movement of fluids away from the legs and towards the upper vessels in the chest while in zero gravity results in physical changes to the vessel walls themselves. These upper vessels which are now loaded with blood, such as the upper torso and the head and neck, appear to become thicker and more cellular, whereas the areas where unloading occurs, like the legs, begin to waste away. This has a direct impact on the vessel's ability to contract and thus exert pressure, which further compounds the problems. Microscopic studies of muscle and nerve biopsies taken from these parts of the body show that the density of nerve endings that secrete mediators responsible for the diametre of the vessels (a concept we read about in the chapter on marathon running) also reduces which in turn influences the ability of blood vessels to relax. Finally, as fluid shifts occur and the body 'perceives' a higher than normal volume of blood (due to more of it migrating towards the brain), signals are sent to the kidney to excrete fluid from the body in an attempt to correct for this oversupply. In parallel, some research also suggests that the number of circulating red blood cells, the blood components that are responsible for binding and transporting oxygen to our tissues, may also diminish. In reality, these changes are fairly inconsequential while we are floating around in space; it is only upon returning to a gravitational field that these changes become apparent and a once-fit athletic individual can be reduced to a collapsed pile of bones and skin.

Like any other muscle, the heart and its cardiac muscles respond to stresses and adapt to them. The blood volume unloading that impacts astronauts while in space causes a reduction in the mass of the heart, its ability to distend and more importantly its ability to contract. Over the years, studies have revealed that astronauts on board the Russian-built Mir space station and later the ISS have smaller and less dynamic hearts, which has led to long-duration crew members setting aside two to three hours per day to exercise while in space. Not the easiest of contraptions but effective nonetheless, astronauts strap themselves to resistance cycling ergometres and treadmills to try and maintain their aerobic fitness during long-term space missions. Another uniquely absurd machine called the Lower Body Negative Pressure Chamber, and one which I have been personally subjected to whilst at NASA, is a device that envelopes your lower limbs and creates an airtight seal around your waist. The vacuum pump then sucks the air out of your lower torso and limbs and draws blood back into those vascular compartments from the upper regions in an attempt to redistribute blood flow.

We have looked at the physical changes that occur in the cardiac muscle in terms of appearance and function. There are also indications that microgravity may induce rhythmic changes in the heart, causing disturbances to the flow of ions — calcium and potassium being the most prominent ones — which are responsible for electrical waves passing through the myocytes. Astronauts undertaking long and stressful extra vehicular activities or spacewalks have been found to have abnormal looking electrocardiograms (ECGs). Another worrying feature observed in almost a fifth of returning crew members is that their QTc period, which is a particular segment of a person's ECG reading that corresponds to the potential excitability of the heart after an action potential has passed through it, is dangerously lengthened. Under normal conditions, this lengthened QTc can lead to life threatening arrhythmias. If they occur whilst in space, these changes will have a detrimental impact on a mission to Mars.

Hip fractures, or in medical lingo 'fractured neck of femurs', are one of the most common fractures associated with growing old. Even with modern surgical techniques and good quality medical care, these injuries are associated with a mortality rate of more than 20% within one year in many developed countries. One of the principal causes for its prevalence in old age is due to decline in bone quality through the normal process of bone remodelling going wrong. Osteoporosis, which in Greek means porous bones, is a progressive bone disease characterised by a decrease in bone mineral density, deterioration in bone microarchitecture, and alterations in the amount and variety of proteins in the bone. Osteoporosis itself has no symptoms; its main consequence is the increased risk of bone fractures, typically occurring in the vertebral column, ribs, hips and wrist. What, you may ask, is the relevance of this discussion on osteoporosis to the current chapter? Well, putting this in perspective, the average post-menopausal woman experiences around 1–2% of bone loss per year. Astronauts lose the same amount, but instead of annually, they do so per month in space! Thus, spaceflight osteopenia is highly relevant as there is a severe increased risk of fractures on long-duration space flights. Moreover, there are potentially detrimental outcomes of raised calcium concentration in the bloodstream, including kidney stones and cardiac arrhythmias. Just imagine the poor astronaut stepping foot on the red planet and, after being holed up in a small spacecraft for more than seven months, suddenly tripping over the last rung of the ladder due his weakened muscles and then falling over and fracturing his hip due the poor quality of his bones.

Dialing 911 will certainly be of little use from 400 million miles away! In order to understand why this happens and how to mitigate these effects, let us examine the basic physiology behind bone modelling and how our musculoskeletal systems undergo repair.

The 206 bones in the adult skeleton create the framework that houses and protects our vital organs and on which all our muscles hang. Made up of calcium and phosphate and taking up around 14% of our body weight, it is in a constant state of flux and renews itself every seven years. Bone remodelling is a lifelong process whereby mature bone tissue is removed from the skeleton through bone resorption and new bone tissue is laid down through ossification. These processes control the reshaping and replacement of our bones following not only major injuries such as fractures but also micro-damage stresses that occur during normal activity. The remodelling of bone is a constant ballet involving a balance between two antagonistic cell lines. The good guys as it were are called osteoblasts, which secrete and lay down new bone material. The bone chompers, on the other hand, or the cells that break down bone, are called osteoclasts. It is the interaction between these two groups that is responsible for the replacement of bones with fresh strong composites at damaged areas. Relying on complex signalling pathways that occur through the action of hormones such as the parathyroid hormone, growth hormone, steroids and immunological activators, these cells utilise calcium, vitamin D and other cellular composites to produce the composite need for bone restoration.

It is a common mistake to think of bone as an inert substance whose sole purpose is to provide a framework and protection for our internal organs. As well as being one of the most physiologically active parts of our body as can be seen from being in a state of constant repair and renewal, bone is also responsible for the manufacture of a large number of important cell lines, including blood and immune system cells, which occur in the bone marrow. One can think of bone as a smooth hard exterior cortex, which is the mechanical component, and an internal trabecular network, which houses the blood marrow and crosslinks. The relative distribution of these two components vary depending on the type of bone — either 'compact' or 'cancellous'. The osteon, also known as the haversian system, is the basic unit of compact bone as it is made up of concentric layers of bony substance surrounding a central haversian canal containing blood vessels and nerves.

As our bony skeleton adapted to cope with environmental stressors and trauma over many generations of human evolution, it developed a unique way to utilise these dynamic forces to shape its own adaptive processes. It is believed that the load exerted on our bones by the shear stress and loads created via the force of gravity are critical stimuli for the remodelling process. This microscopic haversian system transmits loads of differing vectors through the interior core of the bony substance, thereby modulating the activities of the various cell types. In other words, bones actually mold themselves to best suit the stresses and strains put upon them! In the absence of gravity, these important boneshaping forces are removed and with them the bones also lose their drive to self-repair, leading to significant bone loss. Studies conducted on humans and animals as well as in petri dishes placed on the ISS have repeatedly shown the unloading effect of gravity to be two-fold. First, the ability of osteoclasts to eat away at bone (i.e., the resorption) is markedly increased. The pits, which these cells generate on the surface of the bone, appear larger and deeper. Why this process happens still remains a physiological mystery.

Additionally, the repair ability of osteoblasts appears reduced. Again for reasons that are not fully understood, these cells appear lazy and inefficient when in space. Their movement reduces and the material, which they do eventually lay down, is substandard and prone to defects. Worryingly for astronauts, these defects affect the load-bearing bones, namely the hips, pelvis and spine. Therefore, should an accident occur when they reach home or, worse, on a long journey out to space, their bones will be brittle and prone to life threatening fractures.

Bone, as we have just explained, is primarily weakened by the absence of gravity. Secondarily, its metabolic capabilities (that of manufacturing blood and immune cells in the bone marrow) can also be affected in space due to the impact of radiation which reduces cellular generation. This unfortunately is not the end of the damage to the physiological system during long duration space flight. As we have seen, bone is not an inert substance. As the resorptive capabilities of osteoclasts are increased and more bone is broken down, large amounts of calcium also get released into the bloodstream in a condition called hypercalcemia. Calcium is a fundamental ion in various electrophysiological and biochemical pathways across our body and under normal conditions of health, its level is very tightly controlled by our bodies.

In medical school, we were taught the catchphrase *'bones, groans, moans and stones'*, indicating the various effects that hypercalcemia has on the human body. First, the weakened bones allow calcium to adhere to other soft tissues within the body, like tendons and cartilage, and this calcification leads to pain, inflammation and problems with movement. Second, increased calcium also leads to problems with the gastrointestinal system and is a common cause of abdominal pain due to the creation of peptic ulcers and can lead to nausea and vomiting (hence the groans).

Calcium can affect the neurochemistry of the brain and produce symptoms resembling depression and psychiatric moans.

Lastly and most commonly, the increased load of calcium in the bloodstream raises the concentration of calcium in the renal tubules of the kidney. These small particulates can get stuck as they move across the various filters and when they grow to a critical size can cause incredibly painful kidney stones, which if left untreated can be life threatening. The bad news is that these stones require surgical intervention in the majority of cases, which will prove difficult to manage when contained within a restricted space such as on board the ISS or without a trained surgeon on Mars. Another effect of raised calcium concentration in the blood, one that is left out of our very helpful medical school catchphrase, is its effect on the heart. In the last chapter, we learnt about the electrical pathways within the heart, the production of excitatory signals and how action potentials spread across the heart. Calcium has a major role in the normal functioning of these electrical signals and can play an even bigger role in its disruption. Hypercalcemia decreases the heart rate, increases contractility of the cardiac myocytes and makes them prone to arrhythmias and sudden cardiac arrests. Therefore monitoring and preventing the build up of calcium in the blood in addition to the dumping caused by increased bone loss is fundamental to the safety of astronauts in space and is one of the main focuses of scientific research in this field in the past decade.

In much the same way that gravitational unloading affects the bones, the same effects appear in our muscles when we are subjected to microgravity. Muscles also require the constant stimulus of force in order to maintain their shape and strength, and just as bodybuilders workout to increase their muscle bulk, conversely astronauts who don't need to use their muscles in space end up losing them. This muscle atrophy can be profound, particularly for the load-bearing antigravity muscles of our body, such as our legs, back and neck. Studies on astronauts have uncovered muscle bulk loss of around 15 to 20% on long-duration space flights aboard the ISS. As expected, reduced muscle strength is correlated with losses in muscle volume, but the magnitude of the changes in muscle strength appears to be almost 30% greater. As mentioned earlier, majority of these losses generally occur in the trunk and the lower body, especially in muscle groups that are active under normal gravity posture and movement. Upper body strength changes are less dramatic than those observed in the lower body as the crew members use their arms to move around on the space station most of the time by pulling themselves across during their weightless state.

In addition to these gross changes in muscle bulk and power, biopsy results have also shown that cellular changes within muscles further compound the problem. For reasons not fully understood, Type 2 muscle fibre is more prone to atrophy compared to slow-twitch Type 1 muscle fibre. Moreover, there are alterations in the biochemical signalling within muscles and downregulation of their neural circuitry, making them weaker and less effective.

To counteract the negative effects of space, particularly those of microgravity, several measures have been employed by astronauts in order to reduce the amount of bone and muscle loss. These range from pharmacotherapies similar to the drugs used by patients suffering from osteoporosis on Earth (in fact much development in osteoporosis knowledge and treatment is owed to the work done by NASA and the international space community) to more aggressive exercise regimes and specialised equipment. Working on the basis that the physiological problems faced by astronauts are due to the lack of forceful impacts which serve as the main stimulus to encourage healthy bone remodelling and muscle building, most of these machines use resistive technologies that make crew members exercise against a work load. From treadmills, cycle ergometres, bench presses and beyond, the ISS actually has a small gym on board where astronauts can work out for almost two to three hours per day in order to mitigate the harmful effects of lack of gravity on their musculoskeletal systems. The last major system I would like to cover which causes the most immediate stress to astronauts as they enter orbit is the vestibular ocular system, otherwise known as the balancing system. It is perhaps one of the greatest coincidences in my life in which I find myself typing these words. Two weeks prior to this time of writing, I was diagnosed with viral vestibular neuritis, a condition that affected the organs responsible for my sense of balance and rendered me bedridden with severe vertigo. And as I lay there with the world spinning around me, unfortunately causing me to suffer from nausea and vomiting on account of my delicate stomach, I sympathised with all those brave men and women who have sat atop a nuclear bomb and literally blasted themselves into space. For in more than a quarter of all the people who enter low earth orbit, the symptoms of space motion sickness occur. And unlike sea sickness which can be controlled as soon as the boat is docked on dry land, there is no way to remove this effect until their bodies naturally become habituated with the new sensation. Why this happens we shall now examine in more detail.

As we have seen time and time again through this book, the human body is much more intricate and complicated than first meets the eye. Almost constantly across multiple systems, the body builds checks and counter checks to ensure that normal homeostatic mechanisms are in place and working well. Our system of balance which regulates how the body perceives and responds to movement is just one more example of such a mechanism. Our ability to balance is a closely integrated circuit that combines inputs from three main incoming pathways. The largest and crudest of all the signals come from movement sensors called proprioceptors, which we have read about in the previous chapter, located in the large joints like our hips, knees and shoulders. Movements in these joints are sent to the brain to inform it of the direction and speed of these joints in space. Second, our brain receives visual inputs from the world around us which are relayed to the occipital lobe at the back of the brain through the eye. Incoming rays of light falling onto the retina at the back of the eye transmit this data via the optic nerve to the visual cortex located at the rear of our brains. The brain translates this information into an image within our mind, the movement components of which are integrated with the inputs from our joints. Lastly, perhaps the most crucial part of the vestibular ocular system are our specialised organs of balance which reside in our inner ears. This organ, which is barely one centimetre in diametre, is one of the most intricately designed systems in the human body. The inner ear is primarily responsible for balance, equilibrium and orientation in a three-dimensional spatial world and is able to detect both static and dynamic equilibrium. Three semicircular ducts and two chambers which contain the saccule and utricle enable the body to detect deviations from its current resting position. The macula detects vertical acceleration while the utricle is responsible for horizontal acceleration. These microscopic structures possess stereocilia, which are tiny little hairs bathed in a gelatinous membrane. Movements of these hairs caused by the movement of our head enable them to detect motion. The three semicircular ducts on the other hand are responsible for detecting rotational movement and are positioned across different angles so as to achieve a comprehensive view of any changes in position or acceleration.

Upon receiving inputs across all three of these uniquely dynamic and disparate systems, the body integrates these messages into one comprehensive view of itself and its movement in space and this signal creates the sensation of motion. In space, however, gravity is no longer part of the equation and with that, the force required to create fluid shifts within our semicircular canals and inner ears disappear. So while the floating astronaut's eyes receive inputs from the surroundings telling his brain that he is floating and his joints send inputs to the brain about their movements, his ears are having none of it and telling the brain that he is in fact perfectly still. This conflict in internal messaging wreaks havoc on the various integrating nuclei within the brain and triggers nausea and vomiting as well as visual illusions and disorientation much like motion sickness. The good news is that astronauts can adapt to these conflicting stimuli in much the same way that seafarers get used to the motion of the sea. Over time, these signals reduce as spacefarers become accustomed to these messages and slowly feel less and less sick. The prevalence of space motion sickness is particularly high in new space recruits — inflicting almost a third of first time astronauts — and repeat visitors to the ISS are observed to have lesser and lesser symptoms after multiple trips to space. To deal with this problem, crewmembers are treated with oral medications and usually fare well after 48–72 hours.

Like the chapters before, this one relies heavily on human physiology. Dissecting away at the cardiovascular system first followed by the musculoskeletal system and finally the vestibular ocular system, we have learnt about how the absence of gravity affects our frail yet resilient human bodies. We also read about the harmful effects of radiation on our cells and the possible long-term consequences of high exposure through space travel. But something which we often take for granted and a theme that crops up again and again on long term expeditions, particularly one involving extreme danger, is how our minds work and the risk that these missions impose on our mental well-being.

Space really is the one place where nobody can hear you scream. As the absence of mass in a vacuum means that sound waves lack a medium to be transmitted, hence neither can a person's scream no matter how loud it is. Human beings are social creatures; for millennia we have lived in groups and even in today's busy and nucleated world, although we may be absorbed in our own activities and perhaps less interested in the world around us and our peers, the advent of social media and mobile personal telecommunication devices such as mobile phones highlights how much we still desire connecting with others and sharing our views, thoughts, feelings and expressions. It is this fundamental need for human interaction, whether physical or electronic, that is most worrisome about a Mars-bound odyssey that will likely take up to 500 days in space. For a crew of four to six people millions of miles away in a hazardous environment housed in a fragile module and with communication delays of around 40 minutes from Earth, the psychological impact of this mission could outweigh the physical harms of space.

Studies of long-duration crew members, whether on board the ISS or in extreme remote environments like Antarctica, have time and again highlighted the various psychological disturbances that humans face. From mood changes such as anxiety and depression to conflicts in teamwork dynamics, studies have revealed a whole host of behavioural changes that can be catastrophic for long distance missions. Today, as much research is being done to explore the psychological impact of long-duration confinement and remoteness as is being done to explore the physical impact of space travel. Understanding and employing effective teamwork strategies to keep crew members engaged, happy and comforted is as important as dealing with bone and muscle loss. Pre-flight screening and selection plays an ever important role to ensure that the crew of people who will eventually represent humanity on its first voyage to another planet are harmonious and effective. Similarly, a topic which is often whispered in jest but not always taken seriously is the issue of sexual contact between crew members in space. Whether it is physically possible is still not completely known and even if it were so, what impact it would have on crew dynamics and overall morale is unknown. What if a pregnancy were to occur because of this? Whether unwanted (as the case may be for a round trip to Mars) or wanted (maybe one day as humans try to colonise distant planets), we still do not know anywhere near enough about human embryology in microgravity to know what effects the environment of space will have on human fertilisation and the development of an embryo.

I'll end this chapter by looking to the future. Where is this subject domain headed and what are scientists and physiologists doing to make us less vulnerable while in space, physically at least? The obvious answer, but not necessarily the easiest one, is gravity. We take our own food, atmosphere, pressure, fuel and water with us, so why can't we take our own gravity? Hollywood movies have for a long time depicted spaceships housing artificial gravity. For some of them, the science behind them is reasonably clear (such as a large rotating centrifuge-style capsule), while others just refer to 'graviton' molecules or another form of not yet discovered field to create this force within a space vehicle. In reality, a significant amount of work is being done to develop small centrifugal machines that can be housed within the ISS and other longduration space vehicles. An exercising astronaut could in theory expose his or her body to the centripetal effects of such a system pushing the person away from its centre. How large this device can be, how fast it should rotate and just how effective it will be are still being investigated, but it does appear to be the most logical intervention to mitigate the effects of microgravity.

On some level I wish I was born in the previous generation, for they saw first hand a member of their fellow species set foot upon a world beyond our own — what an amazing feeling that must have been! Since then, while we have made tremendous leaps in technology, we have fallen behind in our exploratory ambitions. Since I was a young boy, I have heard the story of how going to Mars is a mere twenty years away; the sad reality is that those twenty years keep getting extended. I hope this account makes a little step towards inspiring you to read more about this incredible area of science and what I believe is the true destiny of mankind — to reach out beyond the confines of our world, our home; to boldly go where no man has gone before. To you all, I wish you these words — *"Live long and prosper!"*

# 5 The Sahara Desert

*"The desert, when the sun comes up... I couldn't tell where heaven stopped and the Earth began."*

— **Aron Ralston, extract from book 'Between a Rock and a Hardplace' Tom Hanks,** *Forrest Gump,* **1994**

---

*"I watch dawn pushing its way into the canyon. It is Thursday, May 1 — day six of my ordeal. I cannot believe I'm still alive. I should have died days ago. Without any task or stimulus, I'm no longer living, no longer surviving. I'm just waiting. I have nothing whatsoever to do. Only in action does my life approximate anything more than existence. Miserable, I watch another empty hour pass by. [B]ut I have to do something, despite the inutility of any action. I reach for my hammer rock. Adrenaline channels into anger, and I raise the hammer, in retribution for what this wretched piece of geology has done to my hand. All I want now is to simply rid myself of any connection to this decomposing appendage. I don't want it. It's not a part of me. I scream out in pure hate, shrieking as I batter my body to and fro against the canyon walls, losing every bit of composure that I've struggled so intensely to maintain. Then I feel my arm bend unnaturally in the unbudging grip of the chockstone."* — An excerpt from the amazing autobiographical account by adventurer — Aron Ralston in his book, Between a Rock and a Hard Place, which tells his story of despair after being stuck in the Grand Canyon for six days, losing 18 kilograms of body weight and more than 25% of blood volume, before having the epiphany to grant himself freedom, and therefore life, by cutting off his right forearm using a pocket knife.

---

London really is one of the most beautiful cities on Earth. Maybe I am biased having grown up there, but there are truly few days that can be as well spent as a late summer's day with a glass of wine at one of her many parks or at a quaint pub along the River Thames. How beautiful it was then to be married on one of those amazing evenings, as Michael Asher and his bride Mariantonietta Peru discovered in 1986. How strange it was too for the retired SAS regiment commander and his Italian-born Arabic photographer wife to find themselves, after only five days of being married, in Mauritania, Africa, to make the first ever West-East crossing of the Sahara desert by camel and on foot! Although my wife and I also chose Africa for our honeymoon, I can't say we were anywhere near as daring at these adventurers, opting instead to spend most of our time lounging on beaches, horse riding through vineyards and eating our way through food trails along South Africa's beautiful Garden Route. After three months in the oasis of Chinguetti, a medieval trading center in northern Mauritania, the couple set off on August 1986. Passing through Mauritania, Mali, Niger, Chad and the Sudan, they finally arrived at the bank of the River Nile at Abu Simbel in southern Egypt in May the following year, having made an unbroken 4,500-mile journey lasting nine months by camel; the first recorded crossing of the Sahara from west to east by non-mechanical means. The feat was lauded by a report in Reuters as *"the last great journey man had still to make."* But given that humans have inhabited the region around the Sahara for many centuries and that the geopolitical problems that plague the region were not as bad compared to today, why then did this adventurous feat take up to only three decades ago to be completed? The desert, as we will learn about in this chapter, is apparently a much harsher environment than many of us truly appreciate.

The English word 'desert' is derived from the ecclesiastical Latin word *dēsertum*, which means 'to abandon'. Before the 20th century, the word desert was often used in the sense of an unpopulated area without any specific reference to aridity or dryness, but today the word is most often used in reference to climate. Almost a third of our planet's surface is desert-like. Dry, barren land with little or no precipitation (i.e., rain) throughout the year, these vast expanses of land include traditional hot spots like the Sahara desert in Africa, the Arabian desert in the Middle East and the Gobi Desert in Asia as well as the less obvious dry lands of the Arctic and the Antarctic, which, as we read in Chapter 2, is incidentally the largest desert on Earth. Deserts are formed by weathering processes whereby large variations in temperature between night and day put strains on the rocks that consequently break up into pieces. Over time, as these rocks break into smaller and smaller fragments and as the strong winds abrade their surfaces making them tinier and smoother, sand is formed. The grains end up as level sheets of sand or are piled high in billowing sand dunes, giving them their characteristic silver screen appearance. But while many people think of deserts as extensive areas of billowing sand dunes because of the big screen, deserts do not always look like this. In fact across the world, only around 20% of deserts are actually sand.

Because of their lack of rainfall, deserts are incredibly difficult places for life to exist, let alone thrive. Any life forms that are capable of surviving in deserts do so because of evolved traits that have made them adept at living with very little amounts of water. Typically receiving less than 10 inches of rainfall each year, desert inhabitants often lose more water through evapotranspiration (a combination of water loss through atmospheric evaporation as well as through the life processes of plants) than they gain from precipitation.

The Atacama Desert is the driest place on Earth, receiving an average rainfall of 1 mm per year. Geographic evidence suggests that the Atacama may not have had any significant rainfall from 1570 to 1971 and the plant forms that exist there are so resilient and specialised that they obtain their moisture from dew and fogs that blow in from the Pacific. Of course, the lack of plants also means that there will be a general absence of animals too and the desert animals that do exist show especially clever adaptations for water conservation and heat tolerance. The camel is a superb example of a mammal that has adapted itself to desert life. Minimising water loss by producing concentrated urine and almost completely dry dung, it is also able to lose almost 40% of its body weight through water loss without dying of dehydration. As we will see through this chapter, our physiological features drastically pale in comparison with these well adapted desert creatures.

But just because the desert is devoid of water and most forms of life does not mean it is of no interest to us. Human beings have survived and lived in deserts for millennia by developing ways to obtain food and water from the harsh environment and passing on this crucial knowledge to successive generations. But why have we tortured ourselves like this? Why suffer under the baking sun and parched for thirst when tribes could have easily migrated out to lush fertile lands elsewhere? Well an unfortunate human characteristic, which at times is just as strong as the instinct to survive, is greed. Deserts are minerally some of the richest places on Earth and many wars have been fought and countless lives lost for its treasures such as gold, mineral ores and oil. But without wanting to cast a pessimistic shadow upon our reading, there also exists the true spirit of human endeavour and our relentless will to push ourselves beyond what we consider to be possible.

Welcome to the world of the Marathon des Sables (MdS), otherwise known as the marathon of the sands. The MdS is a six-day, 251 km ultramarathon, which is the equivalent of running six back-to-back marathons. The rules require runners to be fairly self-sufficient — other than water and a tent to sleep in at night which are provided (what a luxury!), they must bring and carry any other equipment and food they wish to utilise or consume during the run. Such is the popularity of the race that one has to register nearly two years in advance. Over a thousand competitors take part each year in the Sahara Desert in southern Morocco and this race is widely considered to be the toughest foot race on Earth.

While most runners manage to complete the race, some fare worse than they thought they would. Behind the celebrations and congratulations lay the real cost of such a feat. Many runners fall by the wayside every year and some end up dying for their passion. We will unpack the physiological reasons for these defeats and explore how the strongest and fittest are able to sustain themselves through this tortuous terrain. But before we do, it is worth reflecting on the story of Mr. Mauro Prosperi.

A former Olympic pentathlete, Mauro was 39 years old when he attempted the MdS in 1994. On his fourth day of the race, a fierce sandstorm threw him completely off course and he lost his way for ten straight days without food and water. The following words are from an excerpt of an interview he gave with an international broadcasting agency a few years ago.

*"Suddenly a very violent sandstorm began. The wind kicked in with a terrifying fury. A yellow wall of sand swallowed me. I was blinded, I couldn't breathe. The sand whipped my face — it*

was like a storm of needles. I wasn't disoriented, but I had to keep moving to keep from getting buried. Eventually I crouched down in a sheltered spot, waiting for the storm to end. It lasted eight hours. When the wind died down it was dark, so I slept out on the dunes. I woke up very early to a transformed landscape. I didn't know I was lost. I had a compass and a map so I thought I could navigate perfectly well, but without points of reference it's a lot more complicated.

After running for about four hours I climbed up a dune and still couldn't see anything. That's when I knew I had a big problem. When I realised I was lost, the first thing I did was to urinate in my spare water bottle, because when you're still well hydrated your urine is the clearest and the most drinkable. When running the Marathon des Sables you have to be self-sufficient, and I was well-prepared: I had a knife, a compass, sleeping bag and plenty of dehydrated food in my backpack. The problem was water. I would only walk when it was cool, early in the morning and then again in the evening. During the day, when I wasn't walking, I'd try to find shelter and shade.

After a couple of days I came across a marabout — a Muslim shrine where Bedouins would stop when they are crossing the desert. I assessed my situation: it wasn't rosy, but I was feeling alright physically. I ate some of my rations, which I cooked with fresh urine, not the bottled urine that I was saving to drink — I started to drink that on the fourth day. While I was there I saw some bats, huddled together in a tower. I decided to drink their blood. I grabbed a handful of bats, cut their heads and mushed up their insides with a knife, then sucked them out. I ate at least 20 of them, raw — I only did what they do to their prey.

I was very depressed. I was convinced I was going to die and that it was going to be a long agonising death, so I wanted to *accelerate it. I wasn't afraid of dying and my decision to take my own life came out of logical reasoning rather than despair. I wrote a note to my wife with a piece of charcoal and then cut my wrists. I lay down and waited to die, but my blood had thickened and wouldn't drain. The following morning I woke up. I hadn't managed to kill myself. Death didn't want me yet.*

*I took it as a sign. I regained confidence and I decided to see it as a new competition against myself. I became determined and focused again. I put myself in order — Mauro the athlete was back. I needed to have a plan. I walked in the desert for days, killing snakes and lizards and eating them raw — that way I drank, too. I think there are some instincts, a kind of deja vu, which kicks in an emergency situation: my inner caveman emerged.*

*I was aware that I was losing an incredible amount of weight. I was so dehydrated I couldn't urinate anymore. Luckily I had some anti-diarrhoea medicine, which I kept taking. On the eighth day I came across a little oasis. I lay down and drank, sipping slowly, for about six or seven hours. I saw a footprint in the sand, so I knew people couldn't be far."*

Ten days after the sandstorm hit, Mauro was found by a local tribe and taken to the nearest healthcare facility. Weighing in at 16 kilogrammes less than he started, his body had taken a terrible beating. The experience had affected his eyes and liver and it took him almost two full years to recuperate completely. Four years later, he was back at the starting line and since then has completed eight MdS runs and is currently training for a 7,000 km coast-to-coast run across the entire Sahara. A living legend!

As we have read, deserts have high aridity; that is, very low amounts of water. Most of the hot deserts (which I will focus on in this chapter as we have already explored cold physiology in Chapter 2) also have high diurnal temperature variations throughout the day. The daytime high in the Sahara can easily hit the high forties in degrees Celsius and the nighttime low can go as far as 5–10 degrees Celsius. Resident organisms must therefore be capable of regulating their temperature in accordance with very high daytime conditions followed by cold nights. This effect is exaggerated at higher altitudes due to the thinner air. In addition to this large variation in temperature across the day, it is also common to have subtle differences in temperature between the ground surface and the atmosphere a few feet higher. As solar energy strikes the Earth's surface each morning, a shallow layer of air 1–3 centimetres directly above the ground is heated by conduction. Heat exchange between this shallow layer of warm air and the cooler air above it is very inefficient. On a warm summer's day, for example, air temperatures may vary by up to 16.5°C from just above the ground to waist height, making it very difficult for organisms like human beings to adjust our internal temperature settings as there are such large external variations imposed on our bodies.

Thermoregulation is an organism's ability to keep its body temperature within certain boundaries even as the surrounding environmental temperature fluctuates. When we visited the South Pole in Chapter 2, we read about the sophisticated internal controls of our bodies that help to maintain a fairly constant temperature around the homeostatic value of 37 degrees Celsius. This value is vital to us as it is the optimal temperature for the maintenance of important proteins that our internal biochemical reactions depend on. A protein's three-dimensional structure dictates its specificity and therefore its function. Its shape — held together by millions of tiny and weak electrical and atomic bonds, in particular weak-acting hydrogen bonds — is temperature dependent and any deviation from the operational temperature range results in a physical denaturation of the chemical structure and thus an inability to see through its *raison d'etre*. For the purposes of this chapter, hyperthermia or the increase in bodily temperature will be our focus and we will explore the various physiological mechanisms activated by the body in order to keep us as cool as possible. In thermodynamic terms, heat simply refers to the transfer of energy when one body is hotter than the other. A common misconception is that heat is the same as temperature, which is not the case. An object's temperature is the measure of the average speed of the moving particles that exist within it — the energy of these particles is the object's internal energy. When an object is heated, energy is transferred to it, thus causing its internal energy or its entropy to increase. This provides the object's particles with more kinetic energy, making them more 'energetic' which in turn makes the object hotter.

Hyperthermia is officially defined as a body temperature reading greater than 38.3 degrees Celsius. The two most common reasons for hyperthermia are heat stroke, which will be the core concern of this chapter, and adverse drug reactions. As temperature rises, our bodies use a mix of physiological and behavioural mechanisms to reduce heat production and increase heat loss in order to maintain the core temperature within a comfortable range. It may be useful at this point to revisit Chapter 2 (especially if you have not already done so) as the basic principles are very similar to our adaptations for polar climes; the big and obvious difference being that we need to reduce the temperature instead of raising it!

Through our explorations of the human body so far, we have encountered various kinds of biological sensors called receptors which respond to different kinds of stimuli. These are typically neurologically based transducers which, through the action of protein channel gates, allow ions like calcium and sodium to flow into nerve cells, altering their electrical gradients and firing off nerve impulses through the generation of action potentials. The skin forms a protective layer around our body which acts against physical, chemical and thermal environmental challenges. In addition to providing this physical barrier, the skin also serves as a sensory organ that enables the body to detect external stimuli so that appropriate behaviours can be initiated. Thermosensation is one of the sensory modalities of the skin. Our skin contains millions of tiny temperature receptors called transient receptor potential channels which respond to different bands of temperature increases. Running from the dermal layer of the skin via these nerve fibres, the heat pathways make their way along the spinal cord until they reach the parietal lobe in the brain where they converge on the somatosensory cortex. As the temperature rises, the firing rate of these fibres increases, thus informing the brain to modulate physiological changes.

The small pea-sized part of the brain called the hypothalamus sits at the centre of the body's temperature-controlling apparatus. Sensory input fibres across our bodies focus their energies on the posterior part of this gland which, along with information from central thermoreceptors situated within the hypothalamus itself (sensing the internal body temperature via the bloodstream), combine with one another on the anterior portion of the gland called the preoptic area. Exercise and heat stress combined (such as when running the MsD) increases the brain's temperature, thereby also elevating the arterial blood temperature which is sensed by these central receptors. During exercise in hot environments, the cerebral temperature rises in parallel with the core temperature and if prolonged, exhaustion occurs once a critical internal temperature is reached. This suggests that brain temperature may be a dominant factor underlying motor activity or exercise performance in such harsh and extreme conditions. Our internal thermostat works in conjunction with other involuntary and higher nervous system centres to keep the core temperature constant. Some of these responses are involuntary and mediated by the autonomic nervous system, some are neurohormonal and others are behavioural; we will now explore these mechanisms in greater detail.

As discussed in Chapter 2, skin blood flow responses to bodily heating and cooling are essential for physiological thermoregulation. Just as cold climates cause the body to induce vasoconstriction of blood vessels in the skin in an attempt to prevent convective heat loss, exposure to heat such as during intense exercise results in a reflexive vasodilation effect, which augments heat loss. This effect is primarily driven by the sympathetic arm of our nervous systems and is called the active vasodilator system. The amazing thing about this system is that the range of blood flow to the skin can be modulated to the tune of almost zero (during intensely cold weather) to as high as 8 litres per minute, which equates to close to 60% of our cardiac output. The exact mechanism behind this intrinsically simple response has been debated by scientists for decades. This complex interplay is driven by both centrally and locally mediated actions and is one of the most plastic responses seen in our bodies. Increased skin blood flow leads to increased skin blood volume due to the arrangement of venous plexuses close to the skin surface, and thus more circulating blood from our core is exposed to the skin which enables convective heat loss to occur. The cooler blood is then transferred back to the body core, thereby minimising increases in core temperature during exercise and environmental heat exposure.

The chemical players involved in this process are very similar to those used by the body to redistribute blood flow in skeletal muscle during exercise, such as nitric oxide, prostaglandins, and vasoactive intestinal peptides (which we encountered during our marathon run in Chapter 3). There is an internal paradox to consider while we are on this point. Performing muscular exercise is a common way to cause endogenous increases in core temperature and elicit the reflex cutaneous vasodilation. It is important to remember that although exercise causes this reflex, this is separate from the body's response to hyperthermia and raised core body temperature. Under normal temperature, the onset of exercise causes a reflex vasoconstriction in the skin as part of blood flow redistribution from non-working tissues to active skeletal muscle. However, a prolonged period of exercise usually causes sufficient core hyperthermia to elicit the reflex neurogenic vasodilation in the skin. The skin must therefore 'compete' with our active skeletal muscle for blood flow during exercise and thus the response is modified compared with similar levels of hyperthermia in resting humans. This conflict is further exaggerated when we sweat a lot. Our body begins to dehydrate as sweating occurs, especially if profusely, as this reduces our circulating blood volume. When this happens, again the brain shifts the vasodilation trigger further to the right-hand side of the dose response curve, making it occur at a higher core temperature than it would otherwise normally do so. This helps to maintain adequate blood flow to the critical organs and skeletal muscle for exercise to continue unabated.

The second important cooling mechanism is the sweating reflex, otherwise known as perspiration. While many of us think of this as an unwanted, problematic and sometimes embarrassing response from our body (and one that cosmetic companies have successfully created a multi-billion dollar market off ), sweating does serve a very useful function and is critical in allowing us to engage in long periods of exercise and stay cool despite soaring temperatures. Triggered by the same part of the hypothalamus as mentioned earlier, sweating causes a decrease in our core temperature through evaporative cooling at the skin surface. As the high energy molecules evaporate from the skin, energy is absorbed from the body and released, causing the skin and superficial vessels to decrease in temperature. The cooled venous blood then returns to the body's core and counteracts rising core temperatures (as a side note, the same sweat reflex is also triggered during times of emotional stress, but this is limited to our palms, soles, armpits and foreheads). We have on average around three million sweat glands located across our body and the amount of sweat generated is a complex outcome involving our weight, physical fitness, fluid balance, age and other factors. While sweat is mainly made up of water, it also contains other substances such as sodium, potassium, lactate and other trace minerals. During moderate intensity exercise, sweat losses can average up to two litres per hour.

Nerve fibres from the spinal cord make their way into the skin where they wrap themselves around sweat glands in order to modulate their responses. These glands are made up of water channel membrane proteins called aquaporins (particularly sub class 5) which control the movement of water and solutes across cell surfaces and membranes. The main neuronal pathway behind this mechanism is through cholinergic sympathetic nerves that act via a neurochemical modulator known as acetylcholinesterase. This is different from all the sympathetic neurons we have encountered thus far, which principally act via adrenaline as a signalling chemical. Acetylcholinesterase released by these nerve terminals are rapidly processed by enzymes, which then trigger the gland to generate and secrete sweat. In addition to this pathway, some of the chemicals produced locally by cells to increase blood flow also act upon these glands to upregulate the amount of sweat produced. Interestingly, unlike blood vessel dilation, which is a counterintuitive response to exercise, studies have shown that sweating actually begins well before any measurable increase in body temperature occurs. Some studies indicate that this response is triggered within the first 1.5 to 2 seconds of exercise! How this comes about is still being studied, but it is generally believed that a 'central command' centre is involved in exercise — as our brain initiates the activity and begins controlling and contracting the muscles, a signal is sent to other parts of the body which trigger responses to help the body achieve greater efficiency and performance, sweating being one of them. Prolonged exposure to hyperthermia and prolonged exercise in the heat can cause severe water deficits due to profuse sweating, resulting in hypohydration. This water deficit in the body can result in lower intracellular and extracellular volumes and cause plasma hyperosmolality and hypovolemia, both of which will then impair sweating. This unfortunately leads to a vicious feedback loop in the body. As runners continue across the desert plains of the Sahara during the MdS, their body temperatures climb and they begin to sweat profusely to try and correct this. But these runners can also lose up to a couple of litres of body water per hour in this cooling process, thereby reducing their circulating blood volume. As this happens, their ability to sweat is greatly diminished and thus so is their ability to further reduce body temperature. This can lead to a catastrophic rise in their core temperature, sometimes above 40 degrees Celsius, after which loss of consciousness and death can swiftly occur.

Physical training and heat acclimation can help to improve the mechanisms involved in thermoregulation. People who train regularly and are physically active display earlier and more responsive skin blood flow responses (relative to body temperature) compared with individuals who do not exercise as much. A number of studies have shown that regular exercise and heat acclimation both cause a leftward shift in the relationship between skin blood flow and internal temperature such that the onset of vasodilation occurs at lower internal temperatures and exhibits a larger response. The result is greater levels of skin blood flow and sweating (and thus more efficient heat dissipation) for any given level of core hyperthermia and ultimately better survivability in the desert!

Another physiological response that is triggered during times of high body temperature is a change in the rate of internal metabolic activity. We have read about the increased basal metabolic rate which is activated in cold conditions to raise the body's energy consumption. This increased basal metabolic rate is primarily brought about by the production and release of endocrine hormones such as adrenaline and thyroxine and is mediated via hypothalamic pituitary control. In hot conditions, the reverse happens as the body curtails the production of these metabolically active hormones in an attempt control internal heat production. Additionally, there are alterations in behaviour as we gravitate towards cooler environments, such as shaded places. We also find ourselves yearning to just lie down and spread ourselves flat in an attempt to rest and relax. This fatigue or lethargic conditioning is a way to minimise energy expenditure, reduce the amount of heat produced internally and allow heat loss to occur over as much surface area as possible.

Thirst — the craving for fluids — is one of our most primordial and basic of animal instincts that drive us to source fluids and drink. This reflex is essential in maintaining our body's fluid balance and arises when the volume of water or the amount of solutes reaches beyond a comfortable threshold. Failure to replenish our water stores will lead to dehydration and can cause major metabolic imbalances resulting in kidney failure, seizures, coma and death. More than 70% of the Earth's surface is covered by water and it is well believed that life itself began in the ocean depths as biological chemicals bathed in a sea of solutes and energy molecules came together to create the magic of life. Over millennia, the simple single-celled organisms that emerged in the depths of the ocean began to evolve increasingly complex physiological arrangements, giving way to fish, amphibians, reptiles, animals, mammals, primates and finally humans. As a reflection of this evolutionary heritage, our bodies are primarily composed of water — from our blood, cells and tissues to even our bones, water makes up almost 65% of our body weight. Just like the oxygen we breathe, water is crucial for our survival.

Much of the universe's water is actually produced as a byproduct of star formation. When stars are born, a strong explosion of gas and dust accompanies their birth. When this outflow of material eventually impacts the surrounding gas, the shock waves that are generated compresses and heats the gas and water is quickly produced. Water molecules contain one oxygen and two hydrogen atoms connected by covalent bonds (hence the term $H_2O$). A tasteless, colourless and odourless liquid at standard ambient temperature and pressure, it co-exists on Earth with its solid state, ice, its gaseous state, steam or water vapour, and also as snow, fog, dew and clouds. Once again it is worth noting one of the many cosmic coincidences that has created a habitat for life to flourish. Earth is located in a habitable zone within our solar system; that is, if it was slightly closer to or farther away from the Sun (only to the tune of 5% either way), the conditions that enable the three forms of water to exist simultaneously on Earth would be far less likely to exist. Earth's size is also just perfect for water to exist so freely. Any smaller and its reduced gravity would allow water vapour in the atmosphere to float away; any larger and the intense pressure would limit it to ice. Scientists call this phenomenon the 'Goldilocks zone', named after the famous children's story of Goldilocks and the three bears!

Our body comprises somewhere between 55% to 78% water depending on our size. To function properly, around seven litres of water is needed per day to avoid dehydration; the precise amount depends on the level of activity, temperature and humidity. Although most of this intake comes from the food we eat, we still need to consume about 1.5 to 2 litres of water a day under normal conditions to stay healthy. It is vital for humans to be able to maintain fluid levels within narrow ranges, the goal being to keep the interstitial fluid (i.e., fluid outside the cell) at the same concentration as the intracellular fluid (i.e., fluid inside the cell). This condition is called 'isotonic' and occurs when the same level of solutes are present on either side of the cell membrane so that the net water movement across the cell membranes is zero. If the interstitial fluid has a higher concentration of solutes than the intracellular fluid, it then pulls water out of the cell and if enough water leaves the cell, it will then shrivel in dehydration and be unable to perform its essential chemical functions. On the other hand, if the interstitial fluid becomes less concentrated, the cell will fill with water from the outside as it tries to equalise the concentrations. This condition is dangerous if left unchecked as it can cause the cell to swell and rupture. Regulating the thirst reflex, one set of receptors detects the concentration of interstitial fluid while the other set detects the circulating blood volume. Hence, there are essentially two drivers of thirst — one being low volume of water in the body and the other being a high concentration of solutes. As we shall see next, the kidney is a pivotal organ in the regulation of the body's water volume and concentration and has evolved incredibly sophisticated mechanisms to achieve this very simple outcome.

I paused before writing this next segment of the chapter. Renal physiology is arguably the most interesting of all the internal physiological systems in the body, but this also means it is probably one of the most complex. In medical school, weeks of lecturing are dedicated to explaining the various components of this complicated system to budding doctors, and thus I wondered what would be the most efficient means to communicate this next segment to readers. Ultimately deciding that a little bit of knowledge about how the kidneys are structured and do their job in cleaning the blood and creating urine would be important to the reader — so here goes!

Located deep in the abdominal cavity, our two bean-shaped kidneys are typically 12 to 14 centimetres long and weigh around 150 grammes. Situated on each side of the spine, the asymmetry within our abdominal cavities caused by the position of our liver typically results in the right kidney being slightly lower and smaller than the left one. Resting on top of each kidney is the adrenal gland which, as we have seen on so many occasions in this book, is critical for the release of various hormones (chiefly adrenaline) to help our body excel under the most extreme of conditions. Surrounded by a tough fibrous capsule and layers of perinephric fat, the kidney has an entry and exit port called the hilum which allows the renal artery to bring fresh unfiltered oxygenated blood into the organ, the renal veins to carry away deoxygenated blood which is now filtered, and the ureters to bring urine away to the bladder for excretion. For its small size, the kidneys receive an extraordinary percentage of cardiac output — up to 20% — and this number reflects one of the chief responsibilities of these little organs, namely filtration and the production of urine.

The kidney's role in the body cannot be understated. Its chief aim is homeostasis; that is, it strives to maintain the status quo and in so doing regulates our acid-base balance, electrolyte concentrations, fluid volume and blood pressure. The kidney accomplishes these functions both independently and in concert with other organs, particularly those of the endocrine system through the interactions of various hormones. The basic structural and functional unit of the kidney is called the nephron, of which there are close to 1.5 million per kidney. Three relatively simple processes that take place in the nephron — filtration, reabsorption and secretion — accomplish many of the kidney's functions. Filtration is the process by which cells and large proteins in blood are sifted out to produce an ultra-filtrate that eventually becomes urine. The kidneys generate around 180 litres of filtrate each day but also go on to reabsorb a large percentage, thus eventually allowing for the generation of only about 2 litres of urine per day. Reabsorption is the active movement of molecules from the ultrafiltrate back into the bloodstream. On the other hand, secretion is the reverse process in which molecules are expelled from the blood, back into the urine, for excretion through urination.

Each nephron begins at the renal corpuscle, which is made up of two structures called the glomerulus and the Bowman's capsule, creating the initial filtration components of the nephron. Each glomerulus is a tuft of capillaries encased by the Bowman's capsule, which receives its blood supply from a tributary of the renal artery. As the diametre of exit blood vessels from the tuft is comparatively smaller than those of the entry ones, a hydrostatic pressure in the glomerulus is created and this pressure provides the driving force for water and solutes to be filtered out of the blood stream into the space made by the Bowman's capsule. The specialised cells within the glomerulus act as a molecular sieve that allows small proteins, electrolytes and water molecules to pass under the pressure gradient created. About 20% of the blood that enters the renal corpuscle is filtered out and the rest simply passes through the capillary tuft and reenters the renal vein after joining up with other exit vessels from other nephrons. The next part of the nephron is the renal tubule, which is made up of the proximal and distal components of the convoluted tubule and my favourite of all, the loop of Henle. The renal tubule is the portion of the nephron containing the tubular fluid that was filtered through the glomerulus. After passing through the renal tubule, the filtrate then continues into the collecting duct system. The physical properties of the cells that line the length of the nephron change dramatically; consequently, each segment of the nephron has highly specialised functions.

The principal role of the proximal convoluted tubule (the first portion of this tube) is reabsorption. About two-thirds of all the salt, water and solutes are absorbed at this point as well as all the useful proteins, amino acids and glucose. Receiving fresh filtrate from the proximal convoluted tubule, Henle's loop is a 'U'-shaped structure that extends from the proximal tubule to the distal one. It is made up of a thick-walled descending limb and a thin-walled ascending limb and finally empties its altered contents into the distal convoluted tubule. The primary role of Henle's loop is to alter the composition of the filtrate by first absorbing water and then solutes. It does this by indirectly altering the concentration of the surrounding cellular fluid, creating an ever-increasing concentration gradient from the top of the loop until the hair pin 'U' bend at the very base. The descending limb is permeable to water and noticeably less impermeable to salt. As the filtrate descends deeper towards the bottom of the loop, water flows freely out of the descending limb by osmosis until the concentration of the filtrate and interstitium is the same. Unlike the descending limb, the thin ascending limb is impermeable to water and actively pumps sodium ions out of the filtrate, thereby generating the hypertonic interstitium that drives this countercurrent exchange. In passing through the ascending limb, the filtrate within the tubule grows increasingly hypotonic as it loses much of its salt content. This hypotonic filtrate is then passed to the distal convoluted tubule as it makes its way towards the collecting ducts. The cells lining the tubules have numerous energy powerhouse mitochondrial cells to produce enough energy (i.e., ATP) for the active transport of the various ions to take place. Much of the ion transport occurring in the distal convoluted tubule is regulated by various hormones secreted by the kidney and beyond. In the presence of the para-thyroid hormone, the distal convoluted tubule reabsorbs more cal-cium and secretes more phosphate. When aldosterone is present, more sodium is reabsorbed and more potassium secreted. Atrial natriuretic peptide causes the distal convoluted tubule to secrete more sodium.

Finally, the filtrate which has been created by the nephron thus far enters the system of collecting ducts to receive its final piece of fine tuning before it enters the system of ureters to be transported to the bladder as urine. The principal goal of the collecting duct system is to readjust the volume of the fluid, and therefore the amount of water, being excreted by the body. This action is modulated by the antidiuretic hormone (ADH).

Under normal conditions, the collecting duct system is impermeable to water, but it becomes permeable once ADH is secreted. ADH affects the function of aquaporins, membrane proteins that selectively conduct water molecules while prevent-ing the passage of ions and other solutes. As much as 75% of the water from urine can be reabsorbed as it leaves the collecting duct through osmosis, a mechanism that is vital for water con-servation in times of dehydration, such as during hot, desert-like conditions. Thus, the levels of ADH determine whether urine will be concentrated or diluted. Some may wonder why I have spent the last few pages describing the contents of the kidney and its role in water regulation in so much detail. Apart from the academic joy of knowing about this mechanism for the reader, there is also the very pragmatic need to appreciate the role of the kidney as its processes can end up being the difference between life and death in the treacherous and extreme environment of the desert. Knowing about this is important as there may come a time (though hopefully never) when we are faced with a life or death situation and we contemplate drinking our own urine; in much the way some of this chapter's protagonists were faced with. Broadly speaking, one should not drink their own urine. Yes it's true that astronauts do in space, but that is after a significant amount of high tech filtration has been applied to it. A healthy person's urine is about 95 percent water, so in the short term it's very tempting to think one can satiate one's thirst and drink to replenish lost water. However after day two or three, the same excreted solution of waste products, including urea, nitrogen, potassium, and calcium — in the urine — starts to accumulate in the kidneys over and over and begin to impact their filtration ability. Post this point a person risks symptoms similar to those brought on by total kidney failure due to dehydration and a toxic build up of metabolites. Additionally, whilst we think of urine as sterile, most of the time it does contain various microorganisms (even more so when concentrated and unhygienic) and therefore drinking the urine further risks the person to infection. Depending on the environment, an adult can survive up to a week without water and three weeks without food. For that reason the Army Field Manual for Survival lists urine on the 'Do Not Drink' list of fluids, along with fish juices, blood, alcohol and sea-water.

In our normal day-to-day lives, we may take water for granted. But for MdS athletes and their physiological processes, the next homeostatic mechanism I will be writing about is critical. We have already read that many of the actions of the kidney are controlled, or rather modulated, through the actions of various hormones. Secretion and reabsorption can be up or down regulated through the release of hormones from higher control centres in the body. One such feedback loop, which is relevant to this chapter about deserts as it is involved in the control of fluid balance (and therefore blood pressure) in the body, is known as the renin-angiotensin-aldosterone system.

When renal blood flow is reduced, a sign that is perceived by the body as having too little water in our system, cells near the glomerulus in the kidneys secrete renin directly into circulating blood. Renin then carries out the conversion of another enzyme, which is secreted by the liver, called angiotensinogen to angiotensin I. Angiotensin I is subsequently converted to angiotensin II by the enzyme ACE found in the lungs. Angiotensin II is a very powerful vaso-active protein that causes blood vessels to constrict which immediately results in increased blood pressure. Angiotensin II also stimulates the secretion of another hormone called aldosterone from the adrenal glands, which sit atop the kidney. Aldosterone causes the tubules of the kidneys to increase the reabsorption of sodium and water into the blood, which as we have read is through the action of aquaporin molecules in the collecting duct system. This increases the volume of extracellular fluid retained by the body in an attempt to conserve fluid. The amazing thing about the renin-angiotensin-aldosterone system is just how many different components of the body are involved in fine-tuning this parameter, highlighting the importance of fluid dynamics in our normal day-to-day lives. Additionally, because of the numerous touch points in this system, scientists have been able to regulate these various steps through the actions of various chemicals that we consume as tablets, thereby creating powerful tools to combat hypertension, otherwise known as high blood pressure. In fact, ACE-inhibitors and angiotensin receptor blockers are amongst the most widely prescribed drugs globally and have contributed greatly to reducing mortality and morbidity associated with hypertension across the world.

Trekking or indeed marathon running through the desert will cause our internal body temperatures to rise and our water and fluid stores to quickly drop. How these symptoms manifest themselves and develop into life-threatening conditions, we shall now read more about. The first stage in this spectrum is colloquially known as heat cramps. As our bodies sweat in an attempt to cool down the core temperature, a large amount of solutes, in particular salts, are lost in this process. A problem then arises as these salts are important for nerve conduction and muscle contraction. Hence, as the muscles get depleted of sodium and potassium ions, they begin to cramp. This process at this initial stage is easily reversible and involves the subject resting in the shade to bring down his or her temperature and also replenishing lost fluids and solutes through rehydration with isotonic drinks, such as the numerous sports beverages that are commercially available. If this process is not reversed, heat cramps can evolve into a more serious illness called heat stroke. As more fluid and salt is lost, the effects of these losses become more pronounced and the normal physiological processes further deteriorate.

A severe version of heat exhaustion, heat stroke occurs when the body temperature crosses 40 degrees Celsius due to environmental heat exposure or the body's inability to control its internal temperature. Symptoms begin with headaches, dizziness, nausea and vomiting. If left unchecked, this can quickly lead to muscle twitches or severe contractions called clonus, hallucinations, confusion, aggression and eventually unconsciousness. The word 'stroke' is used because of the many neurological symptoms that are present. However, this is not to be confused with the traditional strokes that are due to blockages or bleeds in the blood vessels in and around the brain. The reason we see a significant number of neurologically based symptoms is because of alterations in ionic channel functioning in the nerves due to the denaturation of proteins and loss of electrolytes from sweat loss and rising temperature. It is amazing to think that the body is so dependent upon water that even a 2% drop in fluid levels results in the early signs of dehydration. These symptoms then become increasingly severe as more water loss occurs. Initially the heart and respiratory rates begin to increase to compensate for the decreased plasma volume and blood pressure. As our body tries to conserve water by reducing the amount of sweat we produce, a vicious cycle of rising body temperature begins. At around 5 to 6% water loss, grogginess or sleepiness, severe headaches or nausea and a tingling in the limbs known as paresthesia occurs. With 10 to 15% fluid loss, our muscles may become spastic, the skin shrivels, vision becomes harder to focus and increasingly grey, urination greatly reduces and may become painful, and delirium begins. Losses greater than 15% are usually fatal as our organs fail.

Through the chapters, we have read some personal accounts and descriptions of athletes and travellers whose internal body temperatures soared dangerously. Whether it played a part in Jim Peters' participation at the 1954 Empire Games in Chapter 3 or in Mauro Prosperi's MdS attempt earlier in this chapter, heat stroke is critical and dangerous. Treatment must begin immediately and includes the rapid lowering of body temperature and replacement of lost water and electrolytes. One of the biggest physiological consequences associated with heat stroke is the release of an enzyme called creatine kinase into the bloodstream from damaged muscle cells. This protein has a negative effect on our kidneys which, along with the reduced renal blood perfusion due to the hypovolemia associated with increased sweating, can quickly result in the life-threatening condition known as acute renal failure. There are countless unfortunate stories of athletes exercising in the heat or overexerting themselves, leading to the fatal consequences of acute renal failure secondary to the release of creatine kinase from damaged muscle.

Amazingly though, as we have seen through this book, time and again the human body steps up to the challenge. Yes, while being exposed to the extreme conditions of desert heat can indeed be fatal, the human body has a remarkable ability of adapting itself. Athletes and their scientists have discovered that just as we are able to acclimatise to the low-oxygen environment on Everest and perform remarkably strenuous tasks, so too can we acclimatise to heat and physically push on. Studies have shown that repeated bouts of exercise and physical training in a hot environment can produce a marked improvement in our physiological responses. This improved tolerance is known as heat acclimatisation and manifests as a reduction in the incidence and severity of heat illness symptoms with an increased work output concurrent with decreased cardiovascular, thermal and metabolic strain. Some of the changes we have noted that occur during this process include lower core temperature at the onset of sweating, more efficient heat loss via radiation and convection through the skin capillary network, altered metabolic fuel utilisation, reduced salt loss in sweat production and improved exercise economy. While these changes are all set in place after two weeks of training, we begin to see early signature changes after as little as two to three days! Unfortunately, as with most things in life, if you don't use it you end up losing it. In much the same way, if these changes are reinforced through regular exposure, our body quickly forgets the great adaptations it makes and renders us helpless the next time we are exposed to the heat.

Throughout this chapter we have looked at situations where our body temperatures have risen, in some cases soared, above the natural value. But a word that has not appeared at all throughout our discussion is 'fever'. Most of us associate a rise in temperature with a fever and this is indeed normally the case. However, it is important to state that fever is in fact a different phenomenon altogether and should not be confused with the hyperthermia associated with environmental stress and exercise. In a more traditional sense, fever, otherwise known as pyrexia, is associated with temperature rises above 38 degrees Celsius or around 100 degrees Fahrenheit. It is quite a non-specific and vague symptom which can be associated with diseases from infections to blood clots; from autoimmune conditions to cancer. Typically, the stimulant or trigger for the fever, called a pyrogen, stimulates the secretion of a protein called prostaglandin E2 into the bloodstream which acts upon the hypothalamus, our internal thermostat, to raise the body's temperature. In theory, fever can aid the host's defense capabilities and there are certainly some important immunological reactions that are sped up by temperature such that some pathogens, which have strict temperature preferences, could be hindered. However, there are arguments for and against the usefulness of fever, and the issue remains controversial.

The last topic I thought I should touch on in this chapter on deserts and heat-stressed environments is the future. The future — for mankind and, more importantly, for our home Earth.

As we are all well aware, our thirst for materialistic development has begun to outstrip our planet's ability to sustain itself. The millions of tonnes of fossil fuels we have consumed and dumped onto our fragile planetary ecosystem have started to take effect. Global warming is a reality and has the single biggest ability to impact the way life as we know it exists on our planet. In the last 100 years, the world has warmed by approximately 0.75 degrees Celsius. Each of the last three decades has been successively warmer than any preceding decade since 1850. As well as the many physical changes that rising temperature will have upon the physical environment, there are a host of accompanying negative public health issues. With a rise in air allergens, decrease in air quality and rising ozone levels, respiratory conditions that already affect more than 300 million people with asthma globally will be exacerbated. Higher temperatures will also affect those with cardiovascular conditions, particularly the frail and the elderly. We will witness a rise in the number of natural disasters and changing weather patterns that will reduce the supply of fresh drinking water. It is estimated that there are approximately 600,000 child deaths annually due to diarrheal diseases and this will be compounded by the rise in floods, droughts and famines. Rising temperatures will also produce more fertile breeding grounds for infectious agents, especially water-borne diseases and diseases transmitted via insects, snails or other cold-blooded animals. According to the World Health Organisation, taking into account only a subset of the possible health impacts, and assuming continued economic growth and health progress, climate change is expected to cause approximately 250,000 additional deaths per year between 2030 to 2050 — 38,000 due to heat exposure in the elderly, 48,000 due to diarrhoea, 60,000 due to malaria, and 95,000 due to malnourishment in children.

I may have painted a bleak picture, but I am a perpetual optimist and I personally believe that human beings are capable of achieving great things. After all, as this book has already shown us, even in the face of danger and against the harshness of nature we have beaten the odds and conquered Mt. Everest and the South Pole. Almost 60 years have passed since Yuri Gagarin completed the maiden space flight around Earth and more than 50 years ago two men took that one small step on the Moon. If we can work together to achieve these goals, then surely the human spirit of cooperation and excellence will allow us to create a remedial response for the damage caused over the last few centuries. To turn the clock back on our current unsustainable way of life, and to create a world where we are not dependent on oil and natural gas as well as one where we can live within our means to create a lasting and proud legacy for mankind.

# 6 The Mariana Trench

"*The sea is everything. There is a supreme tranquility. The sea does not belong to despots. On its surface iniquitous rights can still be exercised, men can fight there, devour each other there, and transport all terrestrial horrors there. But at thirty feet below its level their power ceases, their influence dies out, their might disappears.*"

— **Jules Verne, 20,000 Leagues under the Sea, 1870**

*The boom could have signalled death. The impact shook the deep-diving bathyscaphe Trieste as Swiss engineer Jacques Piccard and I reached 30,000 feet — just the beginning of our descent to Challenger Deep, the deepest point in the Mariana Trench off Guam. Only the fact that I realised I'd heard it assured me I was still alive.*

*Our team had been training for the past seven months. We knew what to do. The instruments confirmed everything was OK. The Plexiglas window that had just cracked under the immense weight — 8 tonnes per square inch — was not a pressure boundary.*

*We continued on.*

*The temperature inside dipped to 45 degrees Fahrenheit — only slightly warmer than inside a refrigerator. We were in the perpetual blackness of the abyss, save for the vessel's lights. Given our targeted destination, we expected to see things nobody had seen before. We watched jellyfish and translucent invertebrates with light-generating organs dance past the porthole.*

*Then the bathyscaphe settled on the bottom (around 35,800 feet), releasing a mushroom cloud of white silt. It was as if we were swimming in a bowl of milk. Even after 20 minutes, it never cleared. No photographs of our achievement exist. I wish I could say we had said some profound words, but we just shared a quiet moment.*

*— U.S. Navy Lieutenant Don Walsh, as told to Brooke Morton. January 1960*

Used by seafarers for centuries, the term *fathom* is a measure of depth and is precisely 1.8288 metres, or an easier-to-remember 6 feet. The word *league* however has nothing to do with depth; rather it is a term used to describe distance and was approximated as how far an average man could walk in an hour, roughly 3 miles (roughly 5 kilometres). But even in today's modern world of metric conversions where precision often goes down to the thousandths of a metre, some distances remain unimaginable. Take for instance the depth of the deepest part of our world's oceans. 'Challenger Deep' is located within the Mariana Trench in the Western Pacific Ocean and is a small crescent-shaped valley on the deep sea floor at the southern end. At 36,000 feet (that's 11 kilometres), the water is so deep that at the bottom of the trench, the water column above it exerts a pressure of 1,086 bars (15,750 psi), which is over a thousand times the standard atmospheric pressure at sea level — now that's bone-crushing deep! Putting this into perspective, if Mt. Everest were somehow placed on the bottom of this trench, not only would its summit not even break the water's surface, it would in fact be more than 2 kilometres below it!

The Mariana Trench is formed on the boundary between two tectonic plates. On its eastern edge, the Pacific Plate is thrusted beneath the smaller Mariana Plate that lies on it towards the west.

Tectonic plates are huge chunks of rocks almost 100 kilometres thick at times and at more than 180 million years old, the Pacific Plate is among the oldest in the world. Being so dense due to its extreme age, it has sunk far below the surface and deeper still to the relatively younger Mariana Plate, which it abuts. The trench was first 'sounded' during the Challenger expedition in 1875. As a side note, sounding has nothing to do with sound waves or the echo technology we now use to measure depth. In the old-fashioned way, a rope was thrown off the side of a boat with a lead weight tied to its end, after which the length of the rope was measured to calculate depth. It wasn't until January of 1960 when the first manned descent of Challenger Deep was attempted. Two incredibly brave souls, Naval Officer Don Walsh and the craft designer's son Jacques Piccard, manned the US Navy submersible named Trieste, a two-metre metallic sphere attached to a fifty feet-long buoyancy aid filled with 85,000 litres of gasoline. On 23 January 1960, after a 4 hour and 47 minute descent, she reached the ocean floor. This was the first time a vessel, manned or unmanned, had reached the deepest known point of the Earth's oceans.

From the Mariana Trench and scaling Everest to putting men on the Moon, it almost seemed as though the golden age of adventure and discovery had long been lost. Thankfully more than fifty years later (52 years almost to the day), renowned Hollywood director James Cameron decided to repeat the spectacle, this time attempting a solo descent. Ever since he was a little boy, the ocean deep always captivated Cameron; the movies *Titanic* and *Avatar* were merely a way for him to express his love for the great extremes and the journeys of discovery. Well-versed with deep sea dives in cramped pressurised machines, the director had been to low depths before during his filming of documentaries for the famous cruise liner *Titanic* and the deadly warship *Bismark* for the National Geographic channel. However, this adventure would see him attempt a solo dive in a privately built and funded machine down to a depth no one had been to in decades. We shall be visiting the physics of this environment later on, but just to give you a flavour of the extreme conditions associated with this depth, if the ship were to fail, a hatch to were give way or a panel were to burst, death will be certain within microseconds through a physically crushing implosion.

Finally, after many years of planning, on 26 March 2012, the 57-year-old director climbed through an eighteen-inch diametre hatch into his pressurised sphere to adopt an astronaut-like position lying on his back in the pilot seat. For this attempt, the team had designed a vertical submersible almost 3 storeys tall, which was fully kitted with not only state-of-the-art scientific and research equipment like soil samplers, collection nets and biochemical analysers, but more importantly for him, a whole fleet of 3D video cameras, production equipment and eight feet of bright LED lighting illuminating the field of view up to 30 feet all around to capture the experience in as much detail as possible. Supported by the National Geographic channel, Cameron's journey has been converted into a two-hour documentary that combines incredible underwater footage with his cinematic genius.

He christened his vehicle the *Deepsea Challenger* and the 12-tonne torpedo cruised vertically downwards at a rate of 500 feet per minute. Starting off on a choppy 2 metre-high sea under the sweltering tropical heat in the dark of night, the temperature inside the sphere quickly fell to just above freezing as the penetration of the warm air from above became lesser and lesser below the water's surface. The craft was remarkably built with as much precision and engineering as one would expect from a space launch vehicle. Every aspect of its internal environment was finely monitored from the pressure to the concentrations of oxygen and carbon dioxide, temperature and most important of all the pilot's physiological vitals. Rapidly descending through the water, the ship passed the abyssal zone which is the name given to the level of water beyond which sunlight no longer reaches. At this depth, life must not only tolerate the very cold temperature but also find a way to generate energy without relying on sunlight. It is at this depth where the magical world of physiology, which we take for granted above the water's surface, really reveals its true wonders. Plants that have evolved to generate energy from the thermal heat of underwater springs or from mineral deposits and animals that have evolved bioluminescent organs that make them glow in the dark spring up to amaze us. Spending time examining these creatures will in many ways pave the way for a better understanding of the different realms in which life can evolve, survive and thrive; not only on Earth but farther away on other planets and systems within our solar system or even beyond.

2 hours and 36 minutes later, the submarine was quickly approaching the sea floor. In order to lighten the ship and slow its descent, millions of tiny steel pellets were released from its under belly and the director fired up his reverse thrusters to make a controlled landing on the bottom of Challenger Deep. He then recorded plenty of brilliant and detailed footage for scientists to study for many years to come. He also brought back samples of rocks, sediment and most importantly life from these crushing depths. Who knows what amazing biochemical properties and variants will be discovered from these specimens! Finally after some six hours later, his ship started succumbing to the deep pressure of the hadal zone (named after the realm of Hades, the underworld in Greek mythology). Cameron released the 450-kilogramme iron ballast weights to propel his ship to the water's surface in just under

70 minutes. Only two other men had ever seen or experienced the environment at that depth and never had someone done so on their own. His achievement was incredible in terms of engineering as such a robust and technologically sound ship was created, in terms of filming as the environment was captured in such great detail that it could be used not only for humanity at large to experience and enjoy but also for scientific discoveries to be made, and finally because it encapsulated the spirit of adventure and what it means to be human.

The hero of this chapter, at least at the face of it, is water, and we have met water a few times in this book already, albeit under different guises. A simple yet critical molecule, water really is the stuff of life. In 2008, NASA brought together a team of scientists from across the globe to determine the basic properties a planet needs in order to support life. Top of that list was water! Its unique chemistry of hydrogen and oxygen held together by hydrogen bonds forms the basic scaffolding around which biology occurs. Being present in the universe for over 12 billion years, the same atoms that once made up the stars and gas clouds of the early universe now find themselves within your body and mine. We are essentially stardust — what an amazing thought! Water exists on Earth in all three states and is very stable across a range of temperatures and pressures, and it is the liquid form we are most interested in diving into (pardon the pun) in this chapter.

I mentioned that water was going to be the hero of this chapter, but actually it isn't. It's the medium by which water manifests itself — the real hero of this chapter is pressure. Measured in *Pascals* after the famous French mathematician, physicist and theologian, pressure is the force exerted by or to an object across its surface area. As water has density and therefore weight, it exerts a compressive force in its liquid state upon the objects immersed within it due to the weight of the water 'above' it pushing down on those immersed objects. Therefore, the deeper one dives underwater, the more water there is exerting this force and the greater the pressure acting on one's body. Interestingly, the pressure exerted by water has nothing to do with its volume and everything to do with depth. For instance, a very large but shallow lake will have less pressure than a small but very deep pond. Hence, while the force felt by a dam may be greater when encasing a large shallow lake than a deep pond, a person putting his or her head underwater in both bodies of water will feel the same at the surface, but when submerged at the bottom of either, it is the diver at the bottom of the small pond who will feel significantly worse off! As I was researching for the next section of this chapter, I realised that it could read like a guest list to a fancy 17th century dinner party in Europe. Boyle, Dalton, Henry, Charles, Bernoulli and others are the special guests and the party theme is pressure. It's a whole load of gas (pardon the poor pun, again)! The reason why they are all important in the context of underwater diving is the way gases behave when subjected to depth (i.e., pressure). Take Boyle's law for example, which discusses the inverse nature of the relationship between the volume of a gas and its pressure. Simply put, the deeper one dives, the smaller the volume of gas that amount of air will occupy. This may appear to be unrelated to diving at this stage, but it will make sense when we look at pressure damage in the lungs called barotrauma when a diver ascends too rapidly from depth, causing the delicate air-filled alveoli sacs of the lungs to pop due to sudden rise in volume as pressure is reduced during ascent. And then there is Henry's law, which states that the volume of gas dissolved in a liquid is proportional to the partial pressure of gas above the liquid. Again, this may seem unconnected at first but becomes increasingly important when we look at decompression sickness, also known as 'the bends', when nitrogen dissolved in the bloodstream from the diver's breathing mixture bubbles out of the blood and makes its way into various tissues, causing symptoms as diverse as joint pain and rashes to paralysis and death.

It's tempting to consider underwater diving as a modern sport, with divers using some of the most sophisticated breathing apparatus ever designed. And then there is the older, romantic view of divers being supported by a surface apparatus and supplied with air through long rubber tubes (both of which we shall explore later in the chapter). But a trip through the history of diving actually has stories of divers from many thousands of years ago whose purposes ranged from collecting pearls in Japan over two thousand years ago (this was done by *Ama* divers, who were typically young girls aged 12 to 13 years old wearing an all-white sheer outfit) to military divers as far back as during Alexander the Great's battles (in which divers were used to swim past the enemies' blockade and relay messages to one's allies). Even the ancient Greeks like Plato were indebted to divers who swam to the bottom of the seafloor to collect red coral which was used as a sponge for bathing. And then of course there has always been the more practical and necessary reasons for diving, such as underwater spearfishing.

Fast forward to today and these ancient practices of diving naturally, or unaided, has become known as freediving, which is a form of underwater diving in which divers rely on breath-holding until they resurface rather than the use of breathing apparatus. The name Herbert Nitsch dominates in the global arena as he is commonly known as the 'deepest man on Earth' for his world records. He has over 30 world records across a range of disciplines and the most impressive, at least to me, was the one he achieved in 2012 in Santorini, Greece where, using a weighted device, he reached a depth of 253.2 metres (851 feet). During this dive which lasted more than ten minutes (!), he started to experience symptoms of decompression sickness and upon returning to the surface he was airlifted to a German treatment centre and later suffered a number of strokes. Through extensive rehabilitation he has made a partial recovery, but although he continues to have balance and mobility challenges on land, he still engages in deep freedives. There are of course many great freedivers the world over, some of whom, like Aleix Segura Vendrell of Spain, have achieved records for breath holding for more than 24 minutes (24:03:45 seconds to be exact!). It's just incredible to learn how amazing the body is and what it can do when pushed to the extreme.

When looking at the physiology of diving, a commonly used term is the diving response. Occurring in almost every known air-breathing vertebrate, this response is elicited by apnea (holding one's breath) when submerged in water and consists of peripheral vasoconstriction due to sympathetic nervous system activity and a vagally induced bradycardia with a corresponding reduction of cardiac output. It's exactly the opposite of what happens during running! These changes, brought about by holding one's breath, are further strengthened through a reflex involving the cooling of a person's face (which typically happens underwater), especially around the forehead and eyes. In particularly responsive subjects, apnea has been shown to elevate peripheral circulatory resistance by up to four to five times with correspondingly intense bradycardia and decreased cardiac output. These changes facilitate the supply of blood to a diver's heart and brain.

Our dive reflex also includes two other adaptations, namely the blood shift and the spleen effect. Unlike bradycardia and vasoconstriction, these two additional reflexes occur in response to the increase of water pressure around a diver and not simply to being submerged in water. We encountered Boyle's law earlier and learnt how the pressure of water increases as the diver goes deeper. This increased pressure squeezes a diver's lungs to the extent that when he or she is 100 metres below the surface, the volume occupied by the lungs reduces to around 9% of its original volume! The reason why the rib cage is not crushed at these extremes is because the space created by the reduction in air volume gets occupied by blood and its constituents. Peripheral vasoconstriction causes blood to be shunted towards the central vessels in the chest. As blood travels to the vessels around the alveoli, plasma engulfs these tiny and normally air-filled sacs. As plasma is itself an incompressible fluid, the chest cavity maintains its shape and roughly its size. The second amazing reflex is the splenic effect where the spleen, an otherwise passive organ, begins to contract. Huge volumes of blood normally circulate through the organ as it acts as a reservoir of blood. However, in situations where extra blood is needed, such as during a freedive, the spleen releases blood into the diver's system and then shrinks as blood is emptied. This effect is so great that the Bajau, a group of nomadic people who live in waters winding through the Philippines, Malaysia and Indonesia and who freedive daily to hunt for fish, have spleens almost 50% larger than their mainland cousins.

In 4 B.C., Aristotle first described a diving bell but it was only much later during the 16th century that these bells were made into mechanical aids to augment underwater diving. They are built as rigid chambers that can be lowered into the water and ballasted to remain upright and to sink even when full of air. Oftentimes used to salvage shipwrecks and treasures, earlier versions allowed workers to get around 15 minutes of air, but they still had to work in near pitch-black conditions and were exposed to temperatures as low as 5 degrees Celsius. During the later part of the 17th century, these devices were upgraded to include a fitted window to allow for underwater exploration and had fresh surface air pumped through a system of bellows. Over the centuries, treasure-laden shipwrecks catalysed the development of increasingly sophisticated diving suits consisting of metallic helmets with viewing windows fitted to leather-based airtight suits. The biggest drawback of these systems however remained the constant need to pump surface air into the suits, which restricted the diver's movement and range and was also potentially hazardous as the air supply could get cut off for a number of reasons. It was the Englishman John Lethbridge who first started successfully experimenting in the early 18th century with a process called SCUBA diving, which stands for Self-Contained Underwater Breathing Apparatus and was characterised by an autonomous breathing unit for the diver underwater. The early units were either an open-circuit scuba apparatus where the diver's exhaust was vented directly into the water or a closed-circuit scuba apparatus where the diver's unused oxygen was filtered out from carbon dioxide and recirculated to the diver. However, the compression and storage technology was not advanced enough then to enable compressed air to be stored in containers at sufficiently high pressures such that useful dive times could be achieved. The first commercially available scuba device was tested in 1878 and comprised of a rubber mask connected to a breathing bag, with an estimated 50–60% oxygen supplied from a copper tank and carbon dioxide scrubbed by passing it through a bundle of rope yarn soaked in caustic potash solution. Finally, it was the great wars of the 20th century that led to advancements in both open and closed circuit breathing technologies and produced the modern day equivalents we now use for recreational dive purposes.

It's a very common misconception that our need to breathe is driven by our need for oxygen. Of course, as we have seen on numerous occasions and environments through our journeys together, oxygen is important; nay, critical! But is it the key stimulus for breathing? The answer is no. The real answer lies in carbon dioxide ($CO_2$). We have studied the various receptors in our body that monitor its levels. At elevated states, also known as hypercapnia, the rise in $CO_2$ levels triggers a breathing reflex and raises the respiratory rate. While it is of course true that hypoxia, or low oxygen levels in the blood, also does increase breathing, it is the $CO_2$-mediated trigger that is the more powerful of the two. This is one of the very reasons why you will often see breath-holding divers hyperventilate before a big dive in an attempt to blow out as much $CO_2$ from their lungs (and thus blood) as possible so that the onset of this respiratory trigger is delayed.

Despite being effective in helping divers stay underwater for longer, one problem with this technique is that it increases the risk of a freediving blackout, which is one of the most common causes of drowning amongst this community. A freediving blackout is a loss of consciousness caused by cerebral hypoxia, typically towards the end of a breath-hold dive, when the diver does not experience a need to breathe despite having dangerously insufficient oxygen levels. While there are many causes underlying this phenomenon, the typical sequence of events is a hyperventilation-associated hypocapnia (low $CO_2$ level) which reduces the breathing reflex.

As the diver descends, the higher pressure results in higher partial pressure or concentration of oxygen in the blood which allows the diver to stay down for longer. However, as the diver ascends, the concentration of oxygen reduces alongside the falling ambient pressure and reaches a level low enough for the swimmer to lose consciousness due to insufficient oxygen reaching his or her brain. As we journeyed through the South Pole in the earlier chapter, we learnt about the dangers of cold water immersion, particularly sudden exposure to the cold by falling through an ice sheet and experiencing a cold shock response. The physiological effects described in this chapter are associated with more moderate temperatures and thus changes in physiology are brought on primarily through pressure changes that accompany the process of immersion. Immediate immersion of the body results in changes associated with fluid balance and ventilation. The external hydrostatic pressure of the water causes a blood shift from the extravascular tissues of the limbs into the chest cavity and intravascular space. This perceived increase in blood volume results in a loss of fluids, called immersion diuresis, via the renal system. The shift of blood volume and the enhanced pressure also causes increased respiratory and cardiac workload, of which the effects on the lungs are especially pronounced due to the displacement of the abdominal organs towards the head because of their naturally buoyant state.

A diver's body has two components acting on it: the standard atmospheric pressure and the ambient hydrostatic (water) pressure. A dive descent of 10 metres (roughly 33 feet) in water increases the ambient pressure by an amount approximately equal to the pressure of the atmosphere at sea level. Therefore, a descent from the surface to this depth will roughly result in a doubling of the pressure on the diver. According to Boyle's law, the pressure and volume of gas are inversely related to one another; therefore this pressure change reduces the volume of gas-filled space in the lungs by half.

Barotrauma is a term that is frequently mentioned in diving circles and it refers to tissue damage caused by pressure differences between different compartments of the body. As gas expands due to ambient pressure changes, barotrauma generally manifests as middle ear or sinus effects (seen in up to 30% of divers), decompression sickness, lung tissue injuries and injury to other tissues due to external squeezes caused by raised hydrostatic pressure.

Although descent-based barotrauma due to higher pressures on sensitive areas of the body may sometimes occur, such as cell rupture in the soft tissues of the lung and the small vessels around the eyes, it is ascent-based barotrauma that causes the most common pathologies related to diving. This occurs due to the expanding volume of gas in a closed environment (like the facial sinuses or inner ear) which causes a resultant tension in the surrounding tissues that ultimately exceeds their tensile strength. In addition to cellular and tissue rupture, ascent can also produce gas bubbles and push them into tissues and circulating blood. Catastrophic injuries can ultimately result, including arterial gas embolism, pneumothorax and mediastinal, interstitial and subcutaneous emphysema. The most common reason for such injuries is when divers using compressed gas fail to allow the gas to adequately escape during their ascent phase. As the compressed gas is inhaled at a higher pressure, it begins to expand as the diver ascends. Lungs do not have pain-inducing stretch receptors and thus divers who are not aware of the need to open their airways and exhale through the ascent phase will have little warning before a rupture occurs.

Expanding gas results in air bubbles being produced which can, in many instances, end up in the diver's blood stream. As these bubbles can travel to any part of the body, the symptoms of decompression sickness can vary drastically from joint pains to strokes. To make matters more complicated, individual susceptibility to decompression sickness can also vary from day to day in the same diver. Even different individuals with the same diving history and conditions may be affected differently or not at all. The term 'the bends' was coined to describe the most common manifestation of decompression sickness in roughly 65–70% of cases where gas bubbles make their way to the large joints, such as the shoulders, elbows, ankles and knees. Divers complain of pain in their joints which is aggravated by movement. The next most commonly affected areas are the nerves which account for around 15% of cases and symptoms range from visual disturbances and headaches to more serious effects on the central nervous system, including paresthesia, numbness, seizures, incontinence and paralysis. Manifestations in the skin, such as rashes, itching and swelling, occur in around 10% of cases and are usually not life threatening. There is also a possibility that these bubbles may obstruct blood flow and occluding vessels in both the arterial and venous systems. Bubbles can also injure the vascular endothelium as they move around, resulting in secondary biochemical effects including activation of platelets, immune cells and proteins involved in the clotting cascade.

The final major tissue group affected are the lungs in what is colloquially known as 'the chokes'. Sufferers complain of a dry cough, shortness of breath and pain, typically behind the sternum. Although the onset of decompression sickness can occur rapidly after a dive, symptoms for more than half of all cases typically do not begin to appear until at least one to three hours after resurfacing. In extreme cases, symptoms may occur before the dive has been completed. The risk of a person developing decompression sickness increases when diving for a long period of time or at greater depth. It is also greatly increased if a diver does not follow safety protocols and ascends too rapidly or without making the decompression stops needed to reduce the excess pressure of inert gases in the body. A subtle but important factor that is often overlooked by travelling divers is the risk of developing decompression sickness on the flight home. Commercial aircraft are pressured to an altitude of 2,400 metres (c. 8,000 feet) which greatly increases the risk of gas embolisation in a diver's body if they have not spent adequate time at sea level or have a higher natural risk of decompression sickness. It is therefore advised that divers, particularly those undertaking long or deep dives, spend sufficient time at sea level before embarking on a long flight home. The main culprit in the formation of bubbles is nitrogen (although helium too can lead to decompression sickness). While the location these bubbles initially form is hard to predict, the most likely physical mechanism that underlies bubble formation is a process called tribonucleation, which occurs when two surfaces make and break contact with each other (such as in our joints), and heterogeneous nucleation where bubbles are generated on a surface that is in contact with the liquid. Once the microbubble is formed, their size increases either because of gaseous expansion from the reducing pressure of ascent or by joining with other bubbles in the tissue.

Hippocrates and Homer, two ancient greats, used the word 'narcosis' (from the Greek word *narke*) to describe a 'temporary decline or loss of senses and movement; numbness'. Producing an effect similar to alcohol intoxication, nitrogen narcosis produces an altered but reversible state of consciousness while diving, particularly at depth. Henry's Law states that as pressure rises (such as at depth), the concentration of a gas also increases. As this rising pressure increases the solubility of gases in bodily tissue, gaseous molecules begin to dissolve into the phospholipid membrane of cells, causing direct mechanical interference with and disruption of the transmission of signals between nerve cells. The risk of developing narcosis increases with depth and is most common at dives deeper than 30 metres (100 feet). However, it is also not unusual for a diver's cognition to become affected on dives as shallow as 10 metres (33 feet). Unfortunately, there is no reliable method to predict the depth at which a diver may become struck by narcosis or even the severity of the effect on each individual diver as it can vary from dive to dive even on the same day. While nitrogen is the most common gas from which we see these effects, other inert gases such as argon, krypton and hydrogen can also cause very similar effects. The concentration of a gas required to cause a measurable degree of impairment has been observed to correlate with the lipid solubility of the gas. That is, the greater the solubility, the less the partial pressure of gas needed to create an effect.

One of the nicest rules of thumb I have ever come across concerns estimating the risk of narcosis with depth of diving and is known as Martini's law, or the idea that narcosis results in the feeling that comes with drinking one martini for every 10 metres (33 feet) below a depth of 20 metres (66 feet). Simply put, the mild symptoms of narcosis are similar to that of being a little drunk. At first the diver is welcomed by a sense of calm, confidence and tranquility. These usually remain stable at the given depth and only worsen if the diver goes deeper. As narcosis worsens, divers become more prone to impaired judgement, poorer multi-tasking and coordination, and loss of focus and decision-making ability, which can escalate into a dangerous situation for divers and their group. Other effects include vertigo, visual or auditory disturbances, hallucinations and manic psychological states. Nitrogen narcosis also diminishes the diver's perception of cold discomfort and shivering, thereby affecting the production of body heat and consequently allowing for a faster drop in core temperature in cold water. This condition can be easily overcome by ascending to shallower depths at which the symptoms usually disappear within minutes. If symptoms persist, affected divers are usually expected to abort the dive.

Equivalent narcotic depth is a common way to describe and compare the narcotic effect of different breathing gases. While oxygen and nitrogen are considered to be equally narcotic, hydrogen has a narcotic effect equivalent to half of that of nitrogen (therefore usable to more than twice the depth). Argon however has 2.33 times the narcotic effect of nitrogen and would thus be a very poor choice as a breathing gas for diving. Although helium is the least intoxicating of the breathing gases, it can cause high pressure nervous syndrome at greater depths, which is similar to the other depth-related conditions we encountered earlier that cause a variety of malfunctioning nervous system symptoms, in many cases more extreme.

Sleeping four 'aquanauts', it has an area of 400 square feet with beds, a kitchen, a science lab, bathrooms and a viewing area. Its inhabitants spend days on end conducting medical and scientific experiments in one of the most bizarre environments imaginable. Welcome to Aquarius, a science and research habitat located 6 kilometres off Key Largo at the Florida Keys National Marine Sanctuary. The strange thing about Aquarius is that it is deployed next to deep coral reefs 62 feet (19 metres) below the water's surface. It is the world's premier underwater living habitat as well as NASA's long-term research platform, allowing scientists to remain at the seafloor for extended periods of time. With an ambient pressure 2.5 times greater than that at sea level, visitors to Aquarius have only about 80 minutes to complete their stay and return to the surface before they risk experiencing decompression-related illness. To stay longer, a technique known as saturation diving is employed which allows aquanauts to live and work underwater for days or even weeks at a time. After their missions, aquanauts undergo a 17-hour decompression procedure within Aquarius itself, after which they exit and ascend back to the surface using scuba equipment. The Aquarius habitat and its surroundings provide a convincing analogue for space exploration. Much like space, the undersea world is a hostile, alien place for humans to live.

Our mission to the depths of the oceans has uncovered life in the most exquisite manner and forms, some of which seem thoroughly alien to us and appear better placed on the moons of Saturn than on Earth. With biological adaptations to combat the high pressure, navigate despite complete lack of light and create energy without the sun, these creatures of the deep are bigger, bioluminescent and source their energy from hydrothermal vents on the seafloor. What studying these creatures really teaches us is the resilience of life and its ability to sprout and thrive despite seemingly inhospitable conditions. Most of all, it humbles us as human beings. Despite how amazingly complex and adaptable humans appear to be, there are so many other lifeforms on our own home world that shine a spotlight on how limited our capabilities can be. Known as NEEMO (NASA Extreme Environment Mission Operations), the crew of Aquarius experience some of the same challenges that humans may one day encounter on a distant asteroid, planet or moon. Working in the harsh extreme environments of space and underwater requires extensive planning and sophisticated equipment. This unique environment not only simulates the physical limitations of living on a spacecraft, but also provides the emotional and mental isolation that such missions will involve. What I love most about such amazing human endeavours is how simply they connect two very distinct extreme environments — the expanses of space and the depths of our oceans — and the human pathophysiologies relating to each of them. As our space agencies and an increasing number of private companies plan for manned missions to Mars, asteroids and other satellites within our solar system, analogues like Aquarius allow us to test the limits of our physical, emotional and mental capabilities and develop techniques to keep life at the human edge not merely in survival but also in thrive mode.

# 7 Mitochondria: The Future of Man

*Chapter*

*"Were it not for the melanin in our skin, myoglobin in our muscles and haemoglobin in our blood, we would be the colour of mitochondria. And, if this were so, we would change colour when we exercised or ran out of breath, so that you could tell how energized someone was from his or her colour."*

**— Guy Brown, The Energy Of Life**

It must have been around the third or fourth week of my first year at medical school when we were first introduced to it in so much detail. Starting from the ground up, the first semester of university was spent looking at the cell and all its contents in great depth. I had met it before but not in so much detail. To me, it was merely one part of the whole, an organelle within the cell which, like the other components, worked together to make cells come alive. At the time, that module in cellular physiology was merely a distraction as all I wanted to do was to start learning 'real' medicine — the anatomy and physiology of the heart and the other major organs. Then perhaps I would start to feel like a real medical student and maybe even a doctor. Anyway, study I did and religiously I learned about its structure and chemical nature, how it came to be and its place in our body. There wasn't particularly any enthusiasm or wonder that arose; I did just enough to get through the exams at the end of the year. The word 'mitochondria' would soon get shelved into the recesses of my memory and I got caught up in other more exciting aspects of medical study. But suddenly one day many years later, I heard it again. I was preparing for the Everest expedition and some of the work we were looking at in muscle function and performance at extreme altitudes seemed to be related to the concentration and the efficiency of these tiny organelles. The more I read about them, the more I began to be awed by these tiny structures. It soon dawned on me that mitochondria do not simply exist within us; they serve a much greater purpose in enabling us to do whatever it is that is humanly possible. It also crept up in so many diseases and pathologies, some obscure like those in the footnotes of a chapter on neurological or genetic disorders, but also some major ones that plague so many of us, such as cancer and heart disease. And then we began to see it in the news as scientists found links between mitochondria and ageing and now there are serious discussions as to whether mitochondria could be the Holy Grail in the search for human longevity. Suddenly, studying mitochondria became sexy (to me at least!) and I remember becoming so obsessed with the search for efficiency (the characteristic that makes mitochondria so special) that I once dressed up for a Halloween party as Captain Mitochondria. Although that's a story that makes my wife cringe, I am still proud of that moment!

This chapter can be a little heavier on the science side than some of the previous chapters, but this is aimed particularly at readers who are keen on learning a little more about these tiny but amazing organelles. While we have already met mitochondria at various junctures scattered throughout the book, I will try to provide a broader flavour to the subject with more background detail about mitochondria and how it works while setting the stage for its future and, indeed, ours too.

The first observations of intracellular structures that probably represent mitochondria were published as far back as the 1840s. In 1925, a scientist by the name of David Keilin discovered cytochromes and the respiratory chain was first described. In 1939, scientists demonstrated that cellular respiration using one oxygen atom can form two adenosine triphosphate (ATP) molecules. In 1941, the groundbreaking idea emerged that the phosphate bonds of ATP represent a form of energy currency in cellular metabolism. In the years that followed, the mechanism behind cellular respiration was further elaborated, although its link to mitochondria was still not quite known. As scientific technology developed over time, the ability to isolate these tiny structures improved and cellular respiration was pinpointed as occurring within the mitochondria themselves. The first high-resolution micrographs were taken in 1952 which led to highly detailed analyses of their structure, including confirmation that they were surrounded by a double membrane with the inner one being folded into ridges which divided the inner chamber and that the size and shape of mitochondria varies from cell to cell. Finally in 1976, the genetic and physical maps of yeast mitochondria were completed and that's when the real story began.

The word 'mitochondrion' comes from the Greek word *mitos* meaning 'thread' and *chondrion* meaning 'granule'. They range from 0.5 to 1 micron in size, which is one millionth of a metre, and while their main function as the cellular powerhouse is to generate ATP molecules, they also play a role in cell signalling, cell differentiation, cell cycles and ultimately cell death. The number of mitochondria in a cell can vary widely by organism, tissue and cell type. For example, our red blood cells contain no mitochondria; all of its surface area and volume are dedicated to doing what it does best, which is carrying oxygen. On the other hand, liver cells which have high metabolic demand can have more than 2,000 mitochondrial units per cell. Originating from a bacterial ancestor known as $\alpha$-proteobacteria, mitochondria evolved into endosymbionts (i.e., living inside our cells) over a billion years ago. Lynn Margulis popularised this view of mitochondria's endosymbiotic relationship with host cells when she hypothesised that mitochondria descended from bacteria that managed to survive endocytosis, or being eaten by another cell, and became incorporated into their cytoplasm. The ability of these bacteria to conduct respiration and create energy efficiently would have conferred an evolutionary advantage to host cells that had previously relied on glycolysis and fermentation (both lengthy processes). In turn, host cells evolved to 'tolerate' these aliens and an intimate relationship was formed over the next billion years such that we as the host organism cannot survive without the energy provisions of mitochondria.

Mitochondrial DNA (mtDNA) is a lot smaller than the DNA within our cell nucleus. Composed of a circular format of roughly 16,000 base pairs, it encodes for 37 genes. Mitochondrial genomes have far fewer genes than the bacteria from which they are thought to have descended from. And while some have been lost altogether, many have been transferred to the nucleus itself. This is thought to be relatively common over evolutionary time. Of critical importance is the genetic makeup codes for 13 of the peptides involved in the respiratory chain, which leads to ATP production. Over the past few decades, the classic static and often isolated view of the mitochondrion in the cell has been replaced by an understanding of these organelles living within a dynamic cellular network with close interactions with other components. Mitochondria divide by binary fission. That is, similar with bacterial cell division, they split themselves up into two daughter units. Mitochondrial biogenesis is a complex process that requires the import, synthesis, and incorporation of proteins and lipids into the existing mitochondrial reticulum as well as the replication of the mtDNA. The expression of these genes is regulated by various transcription factors such as NRF-1 and NRF-2 and is modulated by coactivators. As a mechanism to optimise the mitochondrial number and their metabolic capacity, mitochondria biogenesis is activated in response to the imbalance between our energy demands and mitochondrial energy transduction induced by a variety of intracellular signals and extracellular stimuli, such as inflammation. So when the energy needs of our cells are high, mitochondria grow and divide; when energy use is low, mitochondria are destroyed or become inactive. We have already read about the physiological outcomes of these processes in the chapters on Mt. Everest and marathon running.

Our mitochondrial genes are not inherited via the usual mechanism that is responsible for how we inherit the rest of our genes. In humans, when a sperm fertilises an egg cell, the egg nucleus and sperm nucleus each contribute equally to the genetic makeup of the child's zygotic nucleus. However, mtDNA usually comes only from the egg cell. Even though the sperm's mitochondria enter the egg, paternal mitochondria become marked with a protein called ubiquitin which selects them to be destroyed inside the embryo later. So although the egg cell contains relatively few mitochondria, it is only these mitochondria that will survive and divide to populate the cells of the growing fetus. Mitochondria are therefore inherited from mothers, a pattern known as maternal inheritance. This uniparental inheritance leads to almost no opportunity for genetic recombination between different lineages of mitochondria to occur. Any recombination that does take place mainly happens in order to preserve genetic integrity rather than to create genetic diversity. This makes mtDNA a useful source of information for scientists involved in population genetics and evolutionary biology. This unique inheritance pattern has allowed scientists to trace our species lineage through time to arrive at the location of the very first group of human beings — a term biblically known as Adam and Eve. The work of Dr. Allan Wilson has shown that the branches caused by mutations over the millenia converge in a way which makes it clear that our entire species' common ancestor lived in Africa — in northern Botswana. This region, Makgadikgadi, is littered with stone tools dating back almost 2 million years to Homo erectus (a forefather of Homo sapiens). The story being proposed by another expert in the field, Dr. Vanessa Hayes, is that around 200,000 years this region around Lake Makgadikgadi was occupied by our current ancestors — Homo sapiens. For 70,000 years, these people lived in isolation, being penned in by desert conditions around the lake. Then, around 130,000 years ago, due to climatic changes brought upon by changes in the Earth's axis and orbit a green corridor opened up through the deserts, allowing the group to spread out from their 'Garden of Eden' to migrate across the vast plains of Africa and through time populate the entire Earth.

Let us now take a deeper look at the structure of these organelles in order to set the stage for a better understanding of their physiological and biochemical processes. Made up of phospholipids, mitochondria have an inner and outer membrane which divide each unit into five distinct areas. Mitochondrion begins with the two distinct membranes followed by the space between these membranes. The inner membrane is folded in on itself, creating spaces called cristae, and finally there is the internal matrix.

Each of these areas has their own function and process. The outer membrane acts as a checkpoint through which the action of various protein pores called 'porins' allow substances to diffuse in and out of the unit. The membrane is also physiologically active and houses many enzymes involved in metabolic pathways, such as the elongation of fatty acids, oxidation of epinephrine, and the degradation of tryptophan. Thus, the membrane is not a static structure but is instead in continual flux as it interacts with other organelles within the cell. Fusion and fission are continuous events within the cells' interconnected network that regulate not only the mitochondrial morphology but also their biogenesis, transportation, localisation, quality control, degradation and apoptotic cell death. A coordinated balance between fusion and fission serves to maintain the quality of the mitochondrial network. As we shall see later, disturbances to this delicate balance are associated with pathology.

The intermembrane space is the area that exists between the outer and inner membranes. As the outer membrane is permeable to almost all small molecules, the concentrations of small molecules such as ions and sugars in this space end up being the same as the rest of the cell. However, large proteins must have a specific signalling sequence in order to be transported across the outer membrane through the porins, so the protein composition of this space is different from that of the cytosol. One important protein that is localised to the intermembrane space is cytochrome c. The inner membrane is a highly dynamic and metabolically active component that contains many enzymes involved in the oxidative phosphorylation process and ATP synthesis. Unlike the outer membrane, the inner membrane doesn't contain porins and is therefore highly impermeable to all molecules. Almost all ions and molecules require special membrane transporters to enter or exit the matrix. The events of the electron transport chain occur at the inner membrane and because of these movements of electrically charged electrons, a tiny membrane potential is formed which mirrors the resting potential of neurons we read about in Chapter 3 as we visited the South Pole. The inner mitochondrial membrane is folded upon itself to form thousands of cristae which expand the inner membrane's surface area and greatly enhances ATP-producing ability. This structure can increase surface area by almost five-fold in some metabolically active cells like those in the muscles and liver. These folds are studded with small round bodies known as F1 particles or oxysomes. Far from being some simple random folds, these invaginations of the inner membrane can affect their overall chemiosmotic function. First put forward in 1961, the chemiosmostic hypothesis argues that ATP synthesis in respiring cells arises mainly from the electrochemical gradient across the inner membranes of mitochondria, specifically through the energy from NADH and FADH2 as energy-rich molecules such as glucose are broken down. Although controversial at the time, this theory eventually won Peter Mitchell the Nobel Prize in Chemistry in 1978. The theory stated that fuel molecules such as glucose are metabolised to produce acetyl-CoA, an energy-rich intermediate. The oxidation of acetyl-CoA in the mitochondrial matrix is coupled with the reduction of carrier molecules such as NAD and FAD (i.e., electrons are exchanged between them). These carrier molecules then pass the electrons into the electron transport chain on the inner mitochondrial membrane, which in turn pass them on to other proteins further along the chain. The energy in the electrons is then utilised to pump protons from within the internal matrix across the inner membrane, thereby storing up energy in the form of a transmembrane electrochemical gradient which is very similar to the resting potential created in neurons. The protons then move back across the inner membrane down their gradient through an enzyme called ATP synthase, thereby providing the energy for ADP to combine with inorganic phosphate to form ATP. And that is the story of how ATP comes to be in our powerhouse cells. Lastly, the matrix space houses almost 70% of all proteins within these units as well as the machinery required by the units to carry out other functions.

Mitochondria are incredibly clever little organelles. Through the processes of fusion and fission, partially damaged mitochondria can either be rescued by diluting (fusion) or segregating (fission) their damaged components. When severe mitochondrial damage occurs, caused either by energy deprivation, oxidative stress or hypoxia, our cells activate a mechanism that selectively targets and removes these damaged mitochondria. This process, known as mitophagy, includes selective sequestration of damaged mitochondria and their degradation through various receptor-dependent and receptor-independent mechanisms. Several of the mitochondrial functions we have looked at involve a unique interface between the mitochondria and another key organelle in the cell called the endoplasmic reticulum, which produces a structure known as the mitochondria-associated membrane. This is a complex and highly variable structure and contains hundreds of proteins comprising up to 20% of the mitochondrial outer membrane in most of the units. Mitochondria-associated membranes are enriched with enzymes involved in phospholipid exchange, redox homeostasis and calcium signalling. Recent findings have also shown that their functions extend even further to include cellular processes ranging from lipid synthesis and trafficking to calcium signalling, mitochondrial morphology and autophagosome formation.

Damaged and dysfunctional mitochondria have been implicated in a range of human pathologies and the list is steadily growing.

These diseases are as wide-ranging as autism to diabetes and span across myopathies and neuropathies. In majority cases, these diseases are transmitted from the mother to her children as the zygote derives its mitochondria and hence its mtDNA only from the ovum. mtDNA is responsible for syndromes such as KearnsSayre, Pearson and MELAS. Then there are diseases that result from defects in our nuclear genetic material which lead to dysfunctional mitochondrial proteins. This is the case in Friedreich's ataxia, hereditary spastic paraplegia and Wilson's disease. Research conducted over the past decade has also started to implicate the role of these organelles in more common chronic metabolic and lifestyle-related diseases including diabetes mellitus, cardiovascular diseases, Parkinson's disease and Alzheimer's disease. As we have read, the metabolism of lipids and glucose requires mitochondria in order to generate energy. When our consumption of oxygen is lowered due to inefficient nutrient oxidation, there is an increase in the generation of harmful reactive oxygen species. This then impairs different types of molecules, including DNA, lipids, proteins and carbohydrates, leading to pro-inflammatory processes, altered calcium release, protein inefficiency and contractile dysfunction. It is not hard to see that increased uncoupling at the mitochondrial level plays a big part in the emergence of cellular diseases.

As our understanding of mitochondria's role in pathology advances, so too does our knowledge of how we can modulate these effects through genetic and metabolic therapies as well as maximize performance. What has emerged over the past few decades is that cellular metabolism plays a vital role in our ability to perform as well as in our general health and wellness, and pivotal to metabolism is mitochondria. While studies have revealed a strong genetic component underlying an athlete's ability to perform, what is also beginning to surface is the role of the mitochondria and, more specifically, the role of mtDNA in our inherited capabilities for certain skill sets.

mtDNA codes for 13 out of 83 polypeptides in the respiratory chain during ATP production and several studies have highlighted an association between certain mtDNA lineages and performance capability. But how strong this link is and whether it is can be manipulated is still being explored. One of the many ways our body adapts to regular endurance exercise is our skeletal muscles' capacity to utilise oxygen — a rise in the $VO_2$ max — which is the direct consequence of an increased concentration of mitochondrial units. As to how exercise leads to mitochondrial remodelling such that an increase in their number and greater efficiencies are achieved is not clear. Various intermediary transcription factors, such as PGC1a, Allele C and Ser482, or specific genes like the NRF 1 and NRF 2 have been thought to play a role and ongoing studies are looking at how these chemicals express themselves across different population pools and athletic abilities.

As we read in Chapter 3, Kenyan and Ethiopian runners have for the longest time dominated most endurance running events worldwide, from the 5,000-metre track race to the marathon. In fact, almost 70% of the all-time best performances in these events are achieved by Kenyans and Ethiopians. Studies conducted on these populations have demonstrated that the incidence of certain genes within the mtDNA that are thought to be active in endurance athletes were not significantly different between Ethiopian endurance athletes and their general population, whereas the same genes differed between Kenyan runners and the normal population, indicating that in addition to mitochondrial genetic differences and the environment, there may be additional factors which contribute towards creating a champion. Some scientists have also explored the degree of 'coupling' for a person's mtDNA and their corresponding ability to perform physical endurance tasks. Coupling refers to a mitochondrial unit's ability to generate ATP and its efficiency in doing so. It was predicted that people of African descent would have more tightly coupled sets of genes than those of European descent. This would mean that the mitochondria of people of African descent would have the highest ATP production and the lowest heat generation per calorie consumed, making their Type 1 muscle fibres more efficient which then allows them to be better endurance athletes. In contrast, temperate-zone individuals would have less coupled mitochondrial units, therefore although lesser ATP is generated, heat production is higher. Such individuals would be more reliant on Type 2 glycolytic fibres and thus would be more adept at sports requiring short bursts of explosive energy. An increasing amount of preliminary data indicates that this may be the case, although the results are not quite as straightforward as scientists initially predicted. This highlights the complexity of these genomes and how far we are from understanding the physical differences that seem to exist between ethnicities. But these studies also elucidate the importance of nature, the environment and training effects on people's performance and ability. It is also worth noting that the hunt for modulating chemicals that can enhance physical performance is not limited to sports. Militaries around the world are pursuing these biotechnologies in hopes of creating 'super soldiers' — fighters who can perform more effectively on the battlefield while surviving on a low intake of calories. While this may sound like something out of a science fiction movie, it is nonetheless worryingly true.

There are four potential strategies in the endeavour towards greater performance, namely 1. increasing the amount of ATP generated, 2. reducing the amount of harmful free radicals produced, 3. reducing the rate of mitochondrial destruction and 4.

increasing the amount of mitochondrial biogenesis. Once we hit our forties, our muscle mass and strength begin to decline and this degeneration accelerates with advancing age. The loss of muscle mass occurs at a rate of just under 1% per year and appears to be an unavoidable consequence of ageing, although as our work with astronauts in zero gravity has shown, this can be slowed with resistive exercise. While changes such as the accumulation of intramuscular lipids and improper folding of structural and contractile proteins undoubtedly contribute to physical decline, perhaps central to the reducing quality of our muscles is mitochondrial dysfunction. These biochemical changes are accompanied by phenotypic changes in the mitochondria themselves. In old age, a significant proportion of mitochondrial organelles are abnormally enlarged and more rounded in shape. Inside the mitochondria themselves, the mitochondrial cristae and vacuolisation of the matrix are shorter which impairs their ability to create ATP and leads to the production of harmful free radicals, otherwise called reactive oxygen species. Moreover, skeletal muscles cells exhibit a significant decrease in density of mitochondrial units in the elderly. These reactive oxygen species can cause oxidative damage to surrounding structures and the particularly vulnerable mtDNA, resulting in the creation of faulty proteins, oxidised lipids, and mtDNA mutations, all of which contribute to cellular and mitochondrial dysfunction. There is an increasing body of evidence highlighting the role of antioxidants in mopping up these free radicals and preventing them from harming our DNA and cells. Dietary supplements, pharmaceutical remedies or a natural balanced diet with fresh fruit and vegetables are all equally effective ways to boost the presence of antioxidants in our bodies.

One of the most interesting findings in recent years comes from studies showing that most of the declines in mitochondrial function, which are ordinarily attributed to ageing, are instead a result of physical inactivity. When scientists match or control for physical activity levels between young and old subjects, most studies find no age-related changes in mitochondrial enzyme activities, mitochondrial respiration or ATP flux. This is truly astonishing! Interestingly, those studies that do highlight age-related declines tend to involve sedentary young and old people, indicating that these declines in functioning may occur predominantly due to being physically inactive rather than growing old. Increasing evidence points towards our body's ability to turn back the clock at a cellular level by reversing some of the age-related changes on mitochondria with regular exercise. Caloric restriction, which typically involves consuming 20 to 40% fewer calories than normal, can also preserve mitochondrial health and curtail some of the declining functions that accompany old age. Caloric restriction is recognised as the most robust intervention in reducing both primary ageing processes, such as the natural age-related deterioration that occurs in our bodies, and secondary ageing processes, such as accelerated ageing due to disease and unhealthy lifestyle behaviours, thereby potentially increasing our lifespans. Studies carried out by scientists the world over suggest that caloric restriction reduces oxidative stress, facilitates the removal of dysfunctional mitochondria and remodels the body's mitochondrial dynamics such that more fuel-efficient units and less reactive oxygen species are produced.

Over the last hundred years, the field of biochemistry has transformed itself from sitting on the obscure, outer fringes of medicine to being at the forefront of people's minds as pharmaceutical companies and research institutes hunt for the elixir to eternal life. I invite you to imagine a world where the consumption of a syrup can enable athletes to enhance their performance capabilities ten-fold or swallowing a tablet can increase your lifespan by a decade or more; a world where diseases like diabetes and Alzheimer's have been eradicated not through stem cell therapy, the discovery of insulin replacements, or the removal of amyloid plaques in the brain but rather through enhancing the activity of mitochondrial DNA. In such a world, perhaps the topic of mitochondria will no longer be seen as geeky or cryptic and talking about it becomes as ubiquitous and mainstream as the way we speak of hypertension and obesity today. Maybe in that world, the secret life of Captain Mitochondria can be revealed and school kids will dream of donning the magic 'cape of efficiency' or the powerful 'mask of endurance'. Superhero status may very well be a long time away, but I will nonetheless always smile when asked about the great little organelle 'M', and my alter ego's costume will always hang with pride in my cupboard.

# 8 Mind Over Matter

*"I am the happiest man, to run under two hours. In order to inspire many people and tell the world that no human is limited. You can do it!"*

**— Eliud Kipchoge**

Our journey together has been a long one. We have visited the highest mountains, the deepest trenches, the hottest desserts, the coldest poles. We have run farther than any human has run; we have swum deeper than any human has swum. We have even climbed aboard a spaceship and blasted off to visit new worlds in search of life and beauty. But all that while, as our bodies have been pushed to their physical limits — the human edge — there has been an unspoken element which continues to surprise us. In many instances of the stories of heroes, which have appeared throughout this book, the individual faced the very real risks of loss of life or limb. In many instances, this risk was realised. What baffles scientists is the intrinsic ability of the body to perform beyond what the calculated limit should be. Accounting for the survival instinct, even in situations where there is no danger to the loss of life, we see an ability manifests itself which is unexplainable. A source of motivation exists which drives success and achievement in situations in which common sense dictates otherwise. There seems to be a force which makes all these superhuman feats possible.

What takes this complex yet frail biological collection of cells and transforms it to achieve things which excites on-lookers, stuns scientists and inspires generations? What puts the 'be' in human beings? The answer seems to lie beyond the current knowledge of biological systems. Somewhere within the neurochemical circuitry of our physical brains is the generation of this force, this ability. We call this the mind and it is its power over matter which I dedicate the final part of this journey together.

Think about your own experiences. Perhaps you are a runner, a swimmer or a climber. Think back to a time in which you set yourself a target to complete. What happened to you during this journey? Time and time again, in almost every circumstance (and almost always-irrespective of the distance you set yourself), after the halfway mark your body begins to tire and you feel the effort of your task. In most normal individuals, as you achieve 60–70% of the effort, your body begins to slow down as though your mind begins to doubt itself. Post 90% and you can't wait for the target to be reached as you feel yourself performing flat out in an all out effort. Cross the finish line and you feel spent. Does this sound familiar?

Now I would like you to conduct a thought experiment. Imagine you were set the very same distance and completed the task. But as you approached the finish line I sent you a message, maybe as a phone call or a shout, that if you go a further 10% of the distance you stand to gain a prize. Maybe it's money, maybe it's a holiday, a lovely meal or a gold medal. What do you think your response will be? Will you fall off on reaching the finish, like you did before, with no energy left to win the prize? Or will you not only complete the extra 10% but do so with a renewed sense of energy and vigour that you witnessed when you first started the race?

In almost every single experiment conducted around the world looking at this effect, almost every single time we see individuals regain that ability and go on to win the prize. But how is this possible? How did the thought of a gain suddenly negate the physical exhaustion the body was feeling, making it possible to somehow excel?

A study conducted in 2006, which looked at long distance running world records, found exactly the same pattern. In every single instance, in distances beyond 800 metres, a runner's speed would decline up to the 80–90% distance mark, and then suddenly accelerate, at times beating their starting speed. This effect was seen in any distance of effort in every type of condition. Something was influencing the runner, as they seemingly approached their physical limit, to inspire them to break through the barriers and achieve the impossible.

A similar type of study was done in 2014 which looked at 9 million marathon runners(!), from races around the world, spanning four decades, and examined their pacing patterns. Lo and behold the exact same 'U' shaped curve was seen. What was incredible to witness was that at significant hour thresholds (three hours, four hours and five hours), the data showed much higher than expected completion rates immediately before the threshold than immediately after it. This effect was not as strong as half hour splits (three and a half hours, four and a half hours, etc.) and not seen at all for ten minute splits. Something was making the runner speed up as they approached the finish lines, knowing that they were approaching their significant running time threshold. This increase in speed was being achieved even after almost running a full marathon, with all the cruel physiological and metabolic demands we have seen this can have.

Now logic would dictate that the runner is able to anticipate his or her energy needs and pace themselves to create this standard pattern. Knowing that they will require a boost of energy at the end of a race, they hold back a reserve in their tank to spend this to make a strong finish. In some instances this is indeed the case. The same researchers looked at the inflection in speed for various marathon time completion groups and found that the percentage increase was smaller in the three-hour group versus the four-hour or five-hour group. This could indicate that the better trained runners, over the course of their training, learnt how to re-adjust their internal fuel tank and leave less in reserve for the end.

This account is fine, except that we often see this effect in situations like our thought experiment, in which the end goal was extended at the very last moment, or an individual is asked to perform beyond the standard (read expected) end point. How can we then account for this reserve? As it should have already been spent? Or is there an unknown reserve which is effectively a reserve to even our standard reserve which the body keeps in store only for emergency of inspirational prize winning scenarios? That seems unlikely, or does it?

Then there is the story of Diane Van Deren. As a baby of sixteen months, Diane had a prolonged unexpected seizure and was rushed to hospital where she lay convulsing for almost an hour. With no apparent cause found, she grew up into a successful woman with no apparent effects. A star tennis player and mother of two, when she was pregnant with her third child, at the age of twenty-nine, the seizures returned and unfortunately became progressively worse. On the advice of neurologists at the University of Colorado, a partial right temporal lobectomy was performed to remove the focal area of the seizures. What was fascinating about this case is that like other seizure prone individuals, Diane would experience an 'aura' immediately before the event. This manifests itself differently for different people, sometimes as smells, coloured lights, emotions, etc. For her, she found that running would often ward off the seizure. She began doing this, sometimes for hours on end, venturing further and further until she started completing distances like 50 miles, 100 miles, and beyond! She became a running legend and it was Dr. Don Gerber, her neuropsychologist, who first openly speculated that perhaps her amazing physical achievements could have been due to her surgery. It was possible that their lobectomy removed parts of her brain which interprets pain and she does managed it very differently from you or me.

So how is our physical brain anatomy and chemistry linked to this abstract concept of the mind and what is its exact role in endurance?

First proposed in 1924, physiologists hypothesised that the body had a protection system which prevented it from exhausting itself critically. As it became clearer that this limiting factor, fatigue, was not due to the action of peripheral agents like lactic acid, oxygen or fuel depletion — it is increasingly favoured as a 'central' agent in this mechanism. Thus, this theory came to be known as the 'Central Governor' model.

One of the key protagonists of this theorem is a gentleman called Dr. Tim Noakes, a highly influential exercise physiologist. Noakes' hypothesis was that the brain acted as a central governor during a race, limiting our ability to push beyond perceived fatigue to ensure self-preservation, thus effectively over-riding the body's response, slowing us down to preserve physiological health. This signal manifests itself as fatigue giving rise to a subjective feeling that we, as an athlete, have given everything we can. The brain's role, effectively, is to balance the physiological needs to perform, against the need for preservation. The by-product of this is an emotional state which we 'feel' as de-motivation, self-doubt as well as the physical signs of pain.

After all, as Noakes commented on more than one occasion in his research, if physical or aerobic ability was the only influencing factor in achieving success, then assuming that the technique of measuring the underlying mechanisms of VO2max were true (something which we studied in detail in the chapter on running), the Olympic games could be done away with and medals simply handed to the athlete with the highest VO2max score. But as we have seen on so many occasions, the winner is not always the person who is the fittest or the strongest. 'Brainless physiology', in other words, is only half of the picture!

With this in mind, training programs devised for performance now look at 'training the brain' to overcome this restrictive state and allow the body to push forward towards a high level of performance. Brain endurance training is, therefore, a common place technique for athletes looking to enhance their mental will-power and effectively delay the onset of the central governor and its limiting influence on physical ability. Getting used to being bored and overcoming the dullness of pain are important training skills to be learnt, as important as raising one's physical capacity in the pursuit of endurance.

When we visited the South pole together, we learnt about one of the main defence systems our body has — pain. But in all the physiological studies we conducted, around the neurochemical basis of pain and the way it is created and transmitted to the brain, we overlooked a critical part of its role of action. We overlooked its emotional component. We have all suffered before and therefore know that pain is more than just a clinical sign and that, in addition to the physical aspect, it involves an emotional state — a state which can act to either up-regulate or down-regulate the physical part and therefore influencing the outcome. The intense pain of child-birth produces the physiological response to bear down completely, which is then overcome within minutes by the hormonal response to a new born child; the feeling of impending doom associated with the chest crushing pain of a myocardial infarct or angina pectoris; the depressive state of chronic pain syndrome; and the perceived exaggerated response to sometimes undetectable physical ailments. All these are examples of different states of health and sickness and how differently pain, as a symptom, is dealt with.

In evolutionary terms, if your leg was hurt or is bleeding, you would want your brain to shut off the natural signals to stop, especially if you were being chased by a sabre toothed tiger. Stress, fear and anxiety can therefore activate a host of neurohormonal chemicals such as endorphins and endocannabinoids to either dull or completely block out pain which would otherwise overwhelm an individual.

In the same way athletes utilise the subjective feeling of pain to their advantage or disadvantage, harnessing it to push further rather than using it as an excuse to stop. One of the first landmark studies to investigate the perception of pain was conducted by a young graduate student from Scotland in 1981. His hypothesis was to examine the perception of pain amongst different groups of people and he took 30 elite swimmers, 30 club-level swimmers and 26 non-athletes through a protocol designed to measure a person's pain threshold (i.e. giving up), by altering the flow of blood to their forearms. What he found was remarkable. First, the pain threshold was essentially the same in all three groups, i.e. they were all able to complete the same number of exercises when the feeling of pain began. The dramatic difference, however, appeared in their pain tolerance. Elite swimmers were able to complete 132 contractions before giving up; club-level swimmers completed 89; and the non-athletes were only able to manage 70 before calling it quits. Athletes were therefore not 'immune' to pain, but much better at tolerating it and, therefore, able to achieve better results. This difference could be attributed to training, and being 'used to feeling pain' during intense exercise, perhaps due to brain chemicals like endorphins being released to dampen the pain or simply, coming back to our earlier hypothesis, just being better at the psychological coping mechanism of pain. Pain could therefore, in theory, act as a strangely satisfying catalyst to a highly motivated athlete to push themselves further, i.e. it is a stimulus to performance, rather than an inhibitor. Interestingly, the same researcher repeated the studies at three different times of years in the elite athletes and found their scores being the highest during their peak competitive season and lowest in their off-peak season, when they weren't training at all. This profound message is quite startling — that pain in training leads to greater tolerance and subsequently leads to better performance. The old adage of 'no pain, no gain' therefore holds true!

The science that went into Eliud Kipchoge's recent world record feat of running a full marathon in under two hours (1 hour 59.40 seconds) was incredible. From controlling the track and weather conditions, the fuel and hydration inputs, pacing and wind-streaming through a 35-member running team and special shoes designed to enhance efficiency (by 4%), these are all a testament to the amazing work being conducted around the world over by physiologists and researchers to push the body beyond what was thought to be possible. In the end, watching him race past the finish line with the broadest smile on his face that I have ever seen, I couldn't help but wonder how much the mental state that he was in that allowed him to make this physical feat happen. The years of training make it possible for the mind to get used to the signals being sent to it to stop, overcoming the natural feelings of self-doubt, or the boredom of repeatedly putting one foot in front of the other, over and over, thousands of times. Perhaps it was his ability to control his mind in the end, which made the magic happen. And what magic it was!!

So what does all of this mean for us? Perhaps we have to accept that whilst scientists will try and tweak every small known physical variable known to man, we may just need to acknowledge that in the end there is something left unknown, unquantifiable, immeasurable, which keeps taking us right to the human edge, and beyond!

Friends, whatever your journey is, I wish you well. Enjoy it!

# Index

Printed in the United States
by Baker & Taylor Publisher Services